Cardiovascular Emergencies, Part II

Editors

MICHINARI HIEDA
GIOVANNI ESPOSITO

HEART FAILURE CLINICS

www.heartfailure.theclinics.com

Consulting Editor
EDUARDO BOSSONE

Founding Editor
JAGAT NARULA

July 2020 • Volume 16 • Number 3

ELSEVIER

1600 John F. Kennedy Boulevard • Suite 1800 • Philadelphia, Pennsylvania, 19103-2899

http://www.theclinics.com

HEART FAILURE CLINICS Volume 16, Number 3
July 2020 ISSN 1551-7136, ISBN-13: 978-0-323-75452-1

Editor: Stacy Eastman
Developmental Editor: Laura Fisher

Heart Failure Clinics (ISSN 1551-7136) is published quarterly by Elsevier Inc., 360 Park Avenue South, New York, NY 10010-1710. Months of publication are January, April, July, and October. Business and editorial offices: 1600 John F. Kennedy Boulevard, Suite 1800, Philadelphia, PA 19103-2899. Periodicals postage paid at New York, NY, and additional mailing offices. Subscription prices are USD 269.00 per year for US individuals, USD 534.00 per year for US institutions, USD 100.00 per year for US students and residents, USD 300.00 per year for Canadian individuals, USD 618.00 per year for Canadian institutions, USD 315.00 per year for international individuals, USD 618.00 per year for international institutions, and USD 100.00 per year for Canadian and foreign students/residents. To receive student and resident rate, orders must be accompanied by name of affiliated institution, date of term, and the *signature* of program/residency coordinator on institution letterhead. Orders will be billed at individual rate until proof of status is received. Foreign air speed delivery is included in all *Clinics* subscription prices. All prices are subject to change without notice. **POSTMASTER:** Send address changes to *Heart Failure Clinics*, Elsevier Health Sciences Division, Subscription Customer Service, 3251 Riverport Lane, Maryland Heights, MO 63043. **Customer Service: 1-800-654-2452 (US and Canada). From outside of the US and Canada, call 314-447-8871. Fax: 314-447-8029. For print support, E-mail: JournalsCustomerService-usa@elsevier.com. For online support, E-mail: JournalsOnlineSupport-usa@elsevier.com.**

Reprints. For copies of 100 or more of articles in this publication, please contact the Commercial Reprints Department, Elsevier Inc., 360 Park Avenue South, New York, NY 10010-1710. Tel.: 212-633-3874; Fax: 212-633-3820; E-mail: reprints@elsevier.com.

Heart Failure Clinics is covered in *MEDLINE/PubMed (Index Medicus)*.

Contributors

CONSULTING EDITOR

EDUARDO BOSSONE, MD, PhD, FCCP, FESC, FACC
Division of Cardiology, AORN Antonio Cardarelli Hospital, Naples, Italy

EDITORS

MICHINARI HIEDA, MD, MSc, PhD
Assistant Professor, Kyushu University, School of Medicine, Kyushu University Hospital, Fukuoka, Japan; The University of Texas Southwestern Medical Center, Institute for Exercise and Environmental Medicine, Texas Health Presbyterian Hospital, Dallas, Texas, USA

GIOVANNI ESPOSITO, MD, PhD
Professor of Cardiology, University Federico II of Naples, Naples, Italy

AUTHORS

MOHAMMED ALADMAWI, MD
Cardiology Department, Heart Centre, King Faisal Specialist Hospital & Research Centre, Riyadh, Saudi Arabia

BANDAR ALAMRO, MD
Cardiology Department, Heart Centre, King Faisal Specialist Hospital & Research Centre, Riyadh, Saudi Arabia

HANI ALSERGANI, MD
Cardiology Department, Heart Centre, King Faisal Specialist Hospital & Research Centre, Riyadh, Saudi Arabia

CHIARA AMATO
Faculty of Medicine, Federico II University of Naples, Naples, Italy

LUIGI BARBUTO, MD
Department of General and Emergency Radiology, Antonio Cardarelli Hospital, Naples, Italy

MICHELE BELLINO, MD
Cardiology Unit, Cardiovascular and Thoracic Department, University Hospital "San Giovanni di Dio e Ruggi d'Aragona," Salerno, Italy

EWELINE BISKUP, MD
Department of Basic Medical College, Shanghai University of Medicine and Health Sciences, Shanghai, China; Division of Internal Medicine, University Hospital of Basel, University of Basel, Basel, Switzerland

EDUARDO BOSSONE, MD, PhD, FCCP, FESC, FACC
Division of Cardiology, AORN Antonio Cardarelli Hospital, Naples, Italy

ANDREAS BRIEKE, MD
Department of Medicine-Cardiology, University of Colorado Anschutz Medical Campus, Aurora, Colorado, USA

JESSICA BYRD, RN
University of Colorado Hospital, Aurora, Colorado, USA

RODOLFO CITRO, MD, PhD
Cardiology Unit, Cardiovascular and Thoracic Department, University Hospital "San Giovanni di Dio e Ruggi d'Aragona," Salerno, Italy

ANTONIO CITTADINI, MD
Department of Translational Medical Sciences, "Federico II" School of Medicine, "Federico II" University of Naples, Naples, Italy

JOSEPH CLEVELAND, MD
Department of Cardiothoracic Surgery, University of Colorado Anschutz Medical Campus, Aurora, Colorado, USA

ROSANGELA COCCHIA, MD
Division of Cardiac Rehabilitation - Echo Lab, Antonio Cardarelli Hospital, Naples, Italy

WILLIAM K. CORNWELL III, MD
Department of Medicine-Cardiology, University of Colorado Anschutz Medical Campus, Aurora, Colorado, USA

MARTIN CZERNY, MD, MBA, FESC, MEBCTS, FEBVS
Department of Cardiovascular Surgery, Faculty of Medicine, University Heart Center Freiburg, Albert-Ludwigs-University of Freiburg, Freiburg, Germany

SANTO DELLE GROTTAGLIE, MD
Villa dei Fiori, Naples, Italy

PABLO DEMELO-RODRIGUEZ, MD, PhD
Venous Thromboembolism Unit, Internal Medicine, Hospital General Universitario Gregorio Marañón, Sanitary Research Institute Gregorio Marañón, Universidad Complutense de Madrid, School of Medicine, Madrid, Spain

LUIGI DI TOMMASO, MD
Cardiac Surgery Division, Department of Advanced Biomedical Sciences, Federico II University of Naples, Naples, Italy

LORENZO FALSETTI, MD, PhD
Internal and Subintensive Medicine Department, Azienda Ospedaliero-Universitaria "Ospedali Riuniti," Ancona, Italy

FRANCISCO GALEANO-VALLE, MD
Venous Thromboembolism Unit, Internal Medicine, Hospital General Universitario Gregorio Marañón, Sanitary Research Institute Gregorio Marañón, Universidad Complutense de Madrid, School of Medicine, Madrid, Spain

DOMENICO GALZERANO, MD, FESC
Cardiology Department, Heart Centre, King Faisal Specialist Hospital & Research Centre, Riyadh, Saudi Arabia

YOICHI GOTO, MD, PhD
Yoka Municipal Hospital, Hyogo, Japan

RICCARDO GRANATA, MD
Department of Advanced Biomedical Sciences, Federico II University of Naples, Naples, Italy

TOMONARI HARADA, MD
Department of Cardiovascular Medicine, Gunma University, Graduate School of Medicine, Maebashi, Gunma, Japan

MICHINARI HIEDA, MD, MSc, PhD
Assistant Professor, Kyushu University, School of Medicine, Kyushu University Hospital, Fukuoka, Japan; The University of Texas Southwestern Medical Center, Institute for Exercise and Environmental Medicine, Texas Health Presbyterian Hospital, Dallas, Texas, USA

GABRIELE IANNELLI, MD
Cardiac Surgery Division, Department of Advanced Biomedical Sciences, Federico II University of Naples, Naples, Italy

DANIEL KATZ, MD
Fellow in Cardiovascular Medicine, Beth Israel Deaconess Medical Center, Harvard Medical School, Boston, Massachusetts, USA

KENYA KUSUNOSE, MD, PhD, FJCS, FASE, FESC
Department of Cardiovascular Medicine, Tokushima University Hospital, Tokushima, Japan

ALBERTO M. MARRA, MD, PhD
Department of Translational Medical Sciences, "Federico II" School of Medicine, "Federico II"

University of Naples, Centre for Pulmonary Hypertension, Thoraxklinik at Heidelberg University Hospital, Naples, Italy

CIRO MAURO, MD
Cardiology Division, Antonio Cardarelli Hospital, Naples, Italy

RAHUL M. MEHTA, MD
ProMedica Monroe Regional Hospital, Monroe, Michigan, USA

RAJENDRA H. MEHTA, MD
Duke Clinical Research Institute, Durham, North Carolina, USA

MASARU OBOKATA, MD, PhD
Department of Cardiovascular Medicine, Gunma University, Graduate School of Medicine, Maebashi, Gunma, Japan

JAY D. PAL, MD, PhD
Department of Cardiothoracic Surgery, University of Colorado Anschutz Medical Campus, Aurora, Colorado, USA

FILOMENA PEZZULLO, MD
Department of General and Emergency Radiology, Antonio Cardarelli Hospital, Naples, Italy

CHRISTOPHER N. PIERCE, MS, CCP
University of Colorado Hospital, Aurora, Colorado, USA

BRIGIDA RANIERI, PhD
IRCCS SDN, Diagnostic and Nuclear Research Institute, Naples, Italy

PRASHANT RAO, MD
Fellow in Cardiovascular Medicine, Beth Israel Deaconess Medical Center, Harvard Medical School, Boston, Massachusetts, USA

BRETT T. REECE, MD
Department of Cardiothoracic Surgery, University of Colorado Anschutz Medical Campus, Aurora, Colorado, USA

LUIGIA ROMANO, MD
Department of General and Emergency Radiology, Antonio Cardarelli Hospital, Naples, Italy

VALENTINA RUSSO, MD
Department of Advanced Biomedical Sciences, Federico II University of Naples, Naples, Italy

MARWA SABE, MD, MPH
Associate Director of the Advanced Heart Failure Program, Beth Israel Deaconess Medical Center, Harvard Medical School, Boston, Massachusetts, USA

ANDREA SALZANO, MD
IRCCS SDN, Diagnostic and Nuclear Research Institute, Naples, Italy

ANNA AGNESE STANZIOLA, MD, PhD
Section of Respiratory Diseases, Department of Clinical Medicine and Surgery, Federico II University, Centre for Rare Respiratory Diseases, Monaldi Hospital, Naples, Italy

OLGA VRIZ, MD, PhD
Cardiology Department, Heart Centre, King Faisal Specialist Hospital & Research Centre, Riyadh, Saudi Arabia

Contents

Acute myocardial infarction (AMI) results in significant changes in cardiac structure and functions, leading to left ventricular remodeling and subsequent systolic and diastolic dysfunction. To improve current approaches in diagnoses, treatments, and prevention of cardiovascular diseases, a better understanding of cardiac mechanoenergetics, including systolic performance and energy demand, becomes paramount. In this review, we summarize cardiac mechanics, cardiac energetics, and their relationship in complications related to AMI using 2 important physiologic frameworks, pressure-volume loops and the Vo_2-pressure-volume area relationship diagram, as they are powerful tools for understanding physiologic behavior and mechanoenergetics of the left ventricle.

Noninvasive positive pressure ventilation (NIPPV), which can be applied without endotracheal airway or tracheostomy, has been used as the first-line device for patients with acute decompensated heart failure (ADHF) and cardiogenic pulmonary edema. Positive airway pressure (PAP) devices include continuous PAP, bilevel PAP, and adaptive servoventilation. NIPPV can provide favorable physiologic benefits, including improving oxygenation, respiratory mechanics, and pulmonary and systemic hemodynamics. It can also reduce the intubation rate and improve clinical symptoms, resulting in good quality of life and mortality.

The incidence of cardiogenic shock and the utilization of mechanical circulatory support devices are increasing in the US. In this review we discuss the pathophysiology of cardiogenic shock through basic hemodynamic and myocardial energetic principles. We also explore the commonly used platforms for temporary mechanical circulatory support, their advantages, disadvantages and practical considerations relating to implementation and management. It is through the translation of underlying physiological principles that we can attempt to maximize the clinical utility of circulatory support devices and improve outcomes in cardiogenic shock.

biomarker/imaging diagnostic algorithm may help prompt diagnosis and timely treatment along with related improved outcomes. This article describes several clinical cases of cardiovascular emergencies, such as coronary stent thrombosis-restenosis, takotsubo syndrome, acute myocarditis, massive pulmonary embolism, type A acute aortic dissection, cardiac tamponade, and endocarditis.

Clinical Application of Stress Echocardiography in Management of Heart Failure   347

Kenya Kusunose

 Video content accompanies this article at http://www.heartfailure.theclinics.com.

The key to understanding hemodynamics in heart failure (HF) is the relation between elevated left ventricular (LV) filling pressure and cardiac output. Some patients show abnormal response to stress in the relationship between LV filling pressure and cardiac output. In patients with preserved diastolic function, cardiac output can be increased without significantly elevated filling pressure during stress. In patients with HF, as long as the Frank-Starling mechanism operates effectively, cardiac output can increase while acquiring elevated filling pressure. In patients with decompensated HF, hemodynamic stress will lead to a much greater elevation in filling pressure and pulmonary venous hypertension.

Obesity-Related Heart Failure with Preserved Ejection Fraction: Pathophysiology, Diagnosis, and Potential Therapies   357

Tomonari Harada and Masaru Obokata

Obesity is very common in patients with heart failure with preserved ejection fraction (HFpEF). Obesity and increased adiposity have multiple adverse effects on the cardiovascular system, including hemodynamic, inflammatory, mechanical, and neurohormonal effects. Obesity and increased adiposity may be a promising target for therapy in HFpEF. This review summarizes the current understanding of the pathophysiology of obesity-related HFpEF, diagnostic evaluation of HFpEF among obese patients with dyspnea, and potential therapeutic options for the HFpEF obesity phenotype.

HEART FAILURE CLINICS

SERIES OF RELATED INTEREST

Cardiology Clinics
http://www.cardiology.theclinics.com/
Cardiac Electrophysiology Clinics
https://www.cardiacep.theclinics.com/
Interventional Cardiology Clinics
https://www.interventional.theclinics.com/

THE CLINICS ARE AVAILABLE ONLINE!
Access your subscription at:
www.theclinics.com

Preface
Novel Clinical and Pathophysiologic Concepts in Cardiovascular Emergencies

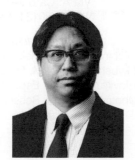
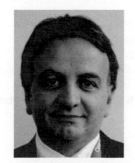
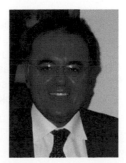

Michinari Hieda, MD, MSc, PhD   Giovanni Esposito, MD, PhD   Eduardo Bossone, MD, PhD, FCCP, FESC, FACC

Editors

Cardiovascular disease (CVD) is a global health problem. A large proportion of clinical manifestations of CVD encompasses cardiovascular emergencies (CE). CE are one of the most common and life-threatening emergencies presenting to the emergency department (ED). Saving time at presentation in ED has always been the cornerstone of CE management. The increasingly rapid evolution in scientific knowledge, technology, and health care system efficiency has critically impacted the field of CE, contributing to saving the lives of patients.

Interestingly, CE can vary in clinical presentation, presenting with either general signs and symptoms typically seen in a wide spectrum of diseases (eg, low/high blood pressure; tachy-/bradycardia) or with some peculiar signs and symptoms that significantly help in the diagnostic process. Indeed, clinical presentations, pathophysiologic mechanisms, and therapeutic options of CE are various and complex, making difficult the systematic collection of CE entities.

As the field of CE is enormous, this issue, "Cardiovascular Emergencies, Part II," focuses on the most common medical problems in CE in the attempt to provide a clinical and pathophysiologic approach to CE from different angles. Specifically, clinical presentation, management, and pathophysiologic mechanisms are presented for acute presentations related to heart failure, aortic diseases, left ventricular assist devices, and pulmonary embolism to mention a few. In addition, common imaging presentation in CE is also presented.

Despite the efforts the current advances in CE management have provided, a lot is needed to grasp the complex reality of CE in clinics. Therefore, we would like to invite the readers of this issue to exercise their critical clinical judgment here, considering the recommendations provided in their own clinical practice as well as in their scientific endeavors.

We believe that a particular strength of this issue is that it brings together the collective efforts of many excellent physicians from diverse clinical specialties. As we all know that dealing with CE is not an easy task, we ensured that the discussion of such complex issues in medicine relied on an international range of authors and institutions in

Heart Failure Clin 16 (2020) xi–xii
https://doi.org/10.1016/j.hfc.2020.04.001
1551-7136/20/© 2020 Published by Elsevier Inc.

heartfailure.theclinics.com

order to provide different, and perhaps complementary approaches, to CE diagnosis, management, and therapy.

All of the efforts of the authors and their collaborators across the globe would not have been possible without the coordination of the Elsevier publishing team to whom goes our sincere gratitude.

Michinari Hieda, MD, Msc, PhD
Kyushu University, School of Medicine
Kyushu University Hospital
3-1-1 Maidashi Higashi-ku Fukuoka City
Clinical Research Building B6F
Fukuoka 812-8582, Japan

Giovanni Esposito, MD, PhD
University Federico II of Naples
Via Pansini 5
Naples 80131, Italy

Eduardo Bossone, MD, PhD, FCCP, FESC, FACC
Division of Cardiology
Cardarelli Hospital
Via A. Cardarelli, 9
Naples 80131, Italy

E-mail addresses:
hieda.michinari.0119@gmail.com;
hieda-m@med.kyushu-u.ac.jp (M. Hieda)
espogiov@unina.it (G. Esposito)
ebossone@hotmail.com (E. Bossone)

Cardiac Mechanoenergetics in Patients with Acute Myocardial Infarction

From Pressure-Volume Loop Diagram Related to Cardiac Oxygen Consumption

Michinari Hieda, MD, MSc, PhD[a], Yoichi Goto, MD, PhD[b],*

KEYWORDS

- Acute myocardial infarction • Pressure-volume loop
- End-systolic pressure-volume relation (ESPVR) • Pressure-volume area (PVA)
- Cardiac oxygen consumption • Tension-area relation • Regional work • Hyperkinesis

KEY POINTS

- The pressure-volume (PV) diagram and the Vo_2-pressure-volume area (PVA) relation are powerful frameworks for understanding behaviors and mechanoenergetics of the left ventricle (LV) in acute myocardial infarction (AMI).
- In the LV PV diagram, there are 3 cardiac properties: (1) end-systolic pressure and volume relation (ESPVR), (2) end-diastolic pressure and volume relation (EDPVR), and (3) effective arterial elastance (Ea).
- PVA represents LV total mechanical energy, and is linearly correlated with myocardial oxygen consumption (Vo_2) per beat.
- The slope of the Vo_2-PVA relation indicates oxygen cost of PVA (contractile efficiency) or the reciprocal of the energy transfer efficiency from oxygen to LV mechanical energy.
- Regional work is represented by wall tension-regional area (TA) loop area, and according to the TA loop framework, hyperkinesis of a nonischemic region is ascribed to regional mechanical unloading rather than regional hyper-performance.

INTRODUCTION

Myocardial ischemia and/or infarction causes significant impairment in the most fundamental cardiac functions: systolic and diastolic functions.[1] There are multiple elements in the pathophysiology of myocardial ischemia and infarction, which include local (or regional) myocardial ischemia, global ischemia (due to decreased coronary perfusion pressure), stunned myocardium (after coronary reperfusion), hibernating myocardium (under long-term coronary hypoperfusion), and myocardial necrosis/fibrosis.[2–5] Also, complications of acute myocardial infarction (AMI) include multiple forms of hemodynamic insufficiency, such as acute heart failure, cardiogenic shock,

Funding: Dr M. Hieda was supported in part by the American Heart Association Strategically Focused Research Network (14SFRN20600009-03). Dr M. Hieda was also supported by American Heart Association post-doctoral fellowship grant (18POST33960092) and the Harry S. Moss Heart Trust.
a University of Texas Southwestern Medical Center, Institute for Exercise and Environmental Medicine, Texas Health Presbyterian Hospital, 7232 Greenville Avenue, Dallas, TX 75231, USA; b Yoka Municipal Hospital, 1187-1 Yoka, Yabu-City, Hyogo 667-8555, Japan
* Corresponding author.
E-mail address: y-goto@hosp.yoka.hyogo.jp

Heart Failure Clin 16 (2020) 255–269
https://doi.org/10.1016/j.hfc.2020.02.002
1551-7136/20/© 2020 Elsevier Inc. All rights reserved.

structural complications, left ventricular (LV) remodeling, and chronic heart failure.[6-9] The LV pressure-volume relationship, also known as pressure-volume loop theory,[10-12] and the cardiac oxygen consumption (Vo_2)-pressure-volume area (PVA) relationship[13-15] are extremely useful in understanding the physiology and mechanism of the LV as well as myocardial energy metabolism[16-21] in various pathologies.[22-24] In this review, we summarize a theory of cardiac mechanoenergetics, which describes a relation between cardiac mechanics and cardiac energetics in the setting of AMI and/or its complication by using 2 important physiologic frameworks of the pressure-volume loops and the Vo_2-PVA relationship diagram.[11,12,25,26]

CARDIAC MECHANOENERGETICS AND PRESSURE-VOLUME DIAGRAM
Pressure-Volume Loop Diagram

End-systolic pressure-volume relationship

End-systolic pressure-volume relationship (ESPVR) is defined by the line connecting the left upper corner of multiple pressure-volume (PV) loops under different LV loading conditions (preload and afterload). It provides the maximal LV pressure at any given LV volume, that is, ESPVR represents the LV systolic property.[27-31] The X-intercept of ESPVR is V_0, that is, unstressed LV volume.[32] It is important to note that this relationship is independent of preload and afterload.[33] The slope of ESPVR, end-systolic elastance (Ees), which has been also referred to as E_{max} based on the time-varying elastance model,[27,29] load-independently represents LV contractility, and becomes steeper when ionotropic drugs are used,[33] whereas lesser steep slope is observed with negative inotropic drugs. Because these changes are usually seen with minimum shifts in V_0, Ees and E_{max} are practically interchangeable with each other. The PV loop diagram and fundamental equations related to cardiac properties are shown in **Fig. 1**.

End-diastolic pressure-volume relationship

End-diastolic pressure-volume relationship (EDPVR) is indicated by the LV passive filling curve during diastole.[34,35] The slope of EDPVR signifies the passive LV chamber stiffness, which represents LV diastolic property.[9,36,37] In a low PV range, an increase in pressure is smaller for a given incremental volume. As the LV volume increases to a higher range, the LV pressure also rises more steeply. The elastin fibers, myocytes, and titin molecules in a sarcomere play a role in the process of forming LV stiffness.[38-40] At higher LV

pressure and volume ranges, the collagen fibers and titin are overstretched, resulting in further resistance.[41,42]

Effective arterial elastance

Effective arterial elastance (Ea) is a conceptual framework of total afterload imposed on LV, which integrates arterial stiffness and peripheral arterial resistance, and is calculated by measuring the ratio of ventricular end-systolic pressure to stroke volume (Ea = ESP/SV).[43,44] The interaction between the LV and aorta known as ventricular-arterial coupling is essential in cardiovascular function, and therefore, the ratio of Ea to ESPVR (Ea/Ees) obtained from the PV diagram is often used to elucidate mechanical efficiency and performance of the ventricular-arterial system.[43,45,46]

Stroke work

Stroke work (SW) is defined as external work performed by the LV to eject SV into the aorta during one cardiac cycle, and is measured from the area enclosed by a PV loop[9,47] (**Fig. 2**). SW is

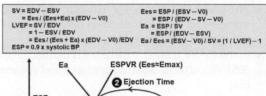

$$SV = EDV - ESV$$
$$= Ees / (Ees+Ea) \times (EDV - V0)$$
$$LVEF = SV / EDV$$
$$= 1 - ESV / EDV$$
$$= Ees / (Ees + Ea) \times (EDV - V0)/EDV$$
$$ESP = 0.9 \times systolic\ BP$$

$$Ees = ESP / (EDV - V0)$$
$$= ESP / (EDV - SV - V0)$$
$$Ea = ESP / SV$$
$$= ESP / (EDV - ESV)$$
$$Ea / Ees = (ESV - V0) / SV = (1 / LVEF) - 1$$

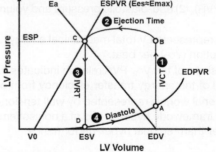

Fig. 1. LV PV diagram. The LV PV loop is delineated by the ESPVR and EDPVR. The slope of ESPVR passes through the ventricular-arterial coupling point (end-systolic volume and pressure) and the volume intercept (V0), which equates to a state of unstressed LV volume. EDPVR represents the LV diastolic property. Ea is depicted with a negative slope connecting between end-diastolic volume and end-systolic pressure point. In a cardiac cycle (in counter-clockwise), *Point A*, the closure of mitral valves (end-diastole); *Point B*, the opening of aortic valves; *Point C*, the closure of aortic valves (end-systole); and *Point D*, the opening of mitral valves. *Duration 1* (from point A to point B), isovolumic contraction time (IVCT); *Duration 2* (from point B to point C), Ejection time (ET); *Duration 3* (from point C to point D), isovolumic relaxation time (IVRT), and *Duration 4*, diastolic time. BP, blood pressure; EDV, end-diastolic volume; ESP, end-systolic pressure; ESV, end-systolic volume; LVEF, left ventricular ejection fraction; SV, stroke volume; V0, unstressed volume (the X-intercept of the ESPVR).

theoretically limited by both ESPVR and EDPVR, but is calculated practically as the product of SV and end-systolic pressure (ESP) during systole (SW = SV $\times$ ESP) by neglecting the diastolic portion.

Potential energy

Potential energy (PE) is measured in the PV diagram as the area enclosed by ESPVR, EDPVR, and the isovolumic relaxation phase segment of a PV loop. PE is residual mechanical energy stored in myocardium at end-systole, which is not released as external work, and is believed to be dissipated as heat during relaxation[15,48] (see **Fig. 2**).

Pressure-Volume area

PVA represents a total mechanical energy generated by the LV contraction during one cardiac cycle,[16,48–50] and consists of SW and PE[48] (see **Fig. 2**). There is a linear correlation between PVA and myocardial oxygen consumption (Vo₂) per beat.[14,22,26,51–55] Because PVA has the dimensions of energy (1 mm Hg·mL = 1.33 $\times$ 10^{-4} J), the concept of PVA can provide a valuable framework to elucidate the LV mechanical efficiency.[19,49,56]

Efficiency of energy transfer

The ratio of SW to PVA is known as LV EET.[57] EET represents the efficiency of mechanical energy transfer from the LV to the arterial system (EET = SW/PVA)[49] (see **Fig. 2**).

Systolic Function

End-systolic pressure-volume relationship in ischemic conditions

There are several theories to describe changes in ESPVR in the setting of global or regional cardiac ischemia.[6,58] The changes seen in the LV systolic and diastolic property from global and local ischemia are shown in **Table 1**. In AMI, LV contractility is decreased, leading to a reduction in stroke volume and blood pressure. The PV loop shifts rightward (initially along the original EDPVR) due to increases in both LV end-diastolic and end-systolic volumes. The global ischemia caused by severe hypoxemia or multivessel coronary artery disease results in generalized hypokinesis of myocardium. This is depicted in the PV diagram as a decrease in Ees with unchanged V₀, resulting in a smaller stroke volume.[59] It is of note that ESPVR may fail to reflect LV systolic dysfunction when LV diastolic pressure is markedly elevated,[60] because ESP is composed of resting diastolic pressure and developed pressure.

On the other hand, in regional ischemia, ESPVR shifts rightward parallel with similar or slightly decreased Ees when compared at a comparable systolic pressure range.[54,61–63] It is challenging to define the behavior of global ESPVR during regional myocardial ischemia. In this setting, it is useful to apply the 2-compartment model; the 2 LV compartments, consisting of ischemic and nonischemic regions, are theorized to be connected through an imaginary conduit that is significantly short in distance.[62] This 2-compartment model may make it easier to understand global function of the LV during regional ischemia. In addition, the parallel rightward shift of the ESPVR during regional ischemia at a comparable systolic pressure range may be partly explained by the nonlinearity of ESPVR during markedly reduced LV contractility[64]

Optimal stroke work and optimal left ventricular efficiency: concept of Qload and Qheart

There have been vast discussions as to whether the LV operates under a condition that maximizes SW or energy efficiency or a combination of the 2 properties. Therefore, the regulatory system is complex with specific combinations of these cardiac properties. Within the framework of the ventricular-arterial coupling, external work (EW) for quasi-isobaric ejection contraction can be estimated as follows:

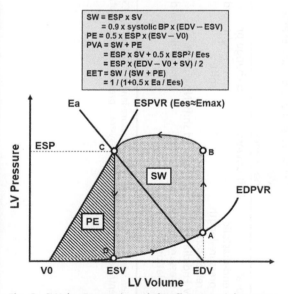

SW = ESP x SV
= 0.9 x systolic BP x (EDV − ESV)
PE = 0.5 x ESP x (ESV − V0)
PVA = SW + PE
= ESP x SV + 0.5 x ESP²/ Ees
= ESP x (EDV − V0 + SV) / 2
EET = SW / (SW + PE)
= 1 / (1+0.5 x Ea / Ees)

Fig. 2. SW (= External work [EW]), potential energy (PE), PVA, and EET. Mechanical work of the LV is composed of SW and PE. The shaded area represents SW, which also equates to EW. SW is calculated by ESP $\times$ stroke volume. The hatched area represents PE. The summation of SW and PE is PVA. PVA is highly correlated with a total oxygen consumption by myocardium. The EET is calculated from SW divided by (PVA = SW + PE). Abbreviations: same as **Fig. 1**.

Table 1
Effect of global and local ischemic change on LV systolic and diastolic property

Category		Global Ischemia		Regional Ischemia	
Systole/Diastole	Local/Global	Severe Systemic Hypoxemia	Severe Systemic Hypotension/Total Coronary Occlusion	Demand Ischemia (Exercise Stress or Pacing)	Supply Ischemia (Coronary Artery Occlusion)
Systolic property	Local myocardium	Fraction shortening ↓	Fraction shortening ↓	Fraction shortening ↓, slope of end-systolic pressure-length relationship (ESPLR) ↓, X-intercept of ESPLR (L0): no change	Fraction shortening ↓↓, ischemic lesion: systolic bulge; non-ischemic lesion: hyperkinesis, ESPLR: rightward shift, X-intercept of ESPLR (L0): ↑
	Global LV	EF ↓↓ (generalized hypokinesis), V0: no change	EF ↓↓ (generalized hypokinesis), ESPVR ↓↓, no change	EF ↓ (regional asynergy), ESPVR ↓, V0: no change	EF ↓ (regional asynergy), ESPVR → or ↓, V0: ↑
Diastolic property	Local end-diastolic pressure-length relationship	Left upward shift	No change or down-rightward shift	Upward shift/working range may move toward right-upward along the new EDPLR	Right-downward shift/working range may move toward right-upward along the new EDPLR
	LV End-diastolic pressure-volume relationship	Left upward shift	No change or down-rightward shift	Upward shift/working range may move toward right-upward along the new EDPVR	Slight right-downward shift/working range may move toward right-upward along the new EDPVR

Abbreviations: EF, ejection fraction; ESPLR, end-systolic pressure-length relationship; ESPVR, end-systolic pressure-volume relationship; L0, X-intercept of end-systolic pressure-length relationship; LV, left ventricle; V0, X-intercept of end-systolic pressure-volume relationship. Up, down, and horizontal arrows indicate increased, decreased, and unchanged, respectively.

$$EW = \frac{Ea}{(1+Ea/Ees)^2}(Ved - V0)^2 \quad (1)$$

where Ved is left ventricular end-diastolic volume (LVEDV) and $V0$ is LV systolic unstressed volume. EW becomes maximum (EWmax) when Ea equals Ees. Substituting Ea with Ees yields EWmax:

$$EWmax = \frac{Ees}{4}(Ved - V0)^2 \quad (2)$$

As the ratio of EW to its maximum value in EW (EWmax), the optimality of the afterload (Qload)[65]:

$$Qload = \frac{4Ea/Ees}{(1+Ea/Ees)^2} \quad (3)$$

The Qload is obtained by equation (1) divided by equation (2), and thus is the function of ventricular-arterial coupling (Ea/Ees) which can vary between 0 and 1. The Qload can become maximum when Ea equals Ees (Ea/Ees = 1). Indeed, in vivo, it has been also reported that the Qload will be maximized under the condition of Ea/Ees = 1.[44,65,66]

Herein, there is another important parameter for the optimality of the heart (Qheart), which requires minimal oxygen per unit time, *but not per beat*, to support the required cardiac work for a fixed afterload. Qheart is defined as follows[66]:

$$Qheart = VO2min/VO2 \quad (4)$$

where Vo_2min is the theoretically estimated minimum oxygen consumption per unit time to generate the required cardiac output within a fixed arterial resistance. When Ved−V0, arterial resistance, and cardiac output are specified, Qheart becomes a function of Ea/Ees. In a theoretic study, the mechanical efficiency per beat is also maximized when Ea/Ees is close to 0.5.[65] Indeed, when Ea/Ees is approximately 0.5 (Ea:Ees = 1:2) in vivo, the cardiac energetics will be most efficient.[66] Therefore, the optimal point for maximum efficiency of Qload and Qheart are similar in a physiologic circulatory system.[65] Interestingly, both Qload and Qheart become close to being most efficient when Ea/Ees is between 0.5 and 1.0, which enables the heart to maximize EW for a given LV preload and minimize the cardiac oxygen consumption, simultaneously.

SW during diastole at a constant PVA does not affect Vo_2. In fact, part of the PE can be converted into SW in an energetically equivalent manner.[67] The LV energy efficiency is close to optimally controlled by baroreceptor reflex under various conditions, but this optimization can fail when contractility decreases.[68] Moreover, both SW and LV energy efficiency are controlled to near optimal levels under various ventricular-arterial coupling conditions.[69] It is also known that LV operates to optimize the EET.[65] In addition, cardiac oxygen consumption (Vo_2) can increase in proportion to Emax while the SW remains constant.[66,70,71]

Diastolic Function

End-diastolic pressure-volume relation under ischemic conditions

Changes in LV EDPVR during myocardial ischemia/infarction are not uniform, depending on the state of coronary flow (maintained or discontinued) and the extent of ischemia (global or regional), and therefore result in multiple forms of pathophysiology and hemodynamic consequences in association with changes in ESPVR (see **Table 1**).[72] Some of them are schematically shown in **Fig. 3**: Cardiogenic shock/low coronary perfusion pressure (see **Fig. 3**A), AMI (see **Fig. 3**B), effort angina (demand ischemia)/heart failure with preserved ejection fraction (see **Fig. 3**C), and post-MI remodeling/advanced heart failure (see **Fig. 3**D). The current understandings of changes in EDPVR in an acute or subacute phase are that (1) EDPVR shifts to the upper-left during hypoxemia (ie, global ischemia/hypoxemia with maintained coronary flow), (2) EDPVR shifts upward during effort angina or pacing-induced ischemia (ie, regional demand ischemia with coronary artery stenosis), and (3) EDPVR is unchanged or may shift to the lower-right when coronary blood flow is reduced (ie, regional supply ischemia with coronary artery occlusion).[70,73–75] In AMI, despite the rightward shift of EDPVR, LVEDP markedly increases in association with decreases in SW and LV dP/dt.[59] This elevation of LVEDP in AMI is explained by a right-upward move of operating range of PV loop along the EDPVR curve due to a decrease in LV systolic function, rather than by a shift of the EDPVR.[59]

Assessment of changes in end-diastolic pressure-volume relation

The nonlinear EDPVR characterizes passive LV diastolic properties reflecting LV chamber stiffness and determines the relationship between LV preload and diastolic filling pressure. There have been several efforts to quantitatively assess EDPVR.[76] Conventionally, EDPVR has been approximated by an exponential function ($P = P_0 \times \{Exp [k (V-V_0)] -1\}$), and its steepness coefficient k is used as an LV stiffness constant.[77] However, it is challenging to accurately approximate EDPVR with an exponential function, because it has been pointed out that the EDPVR is affected by the changes in LVEDP.[77,78] Other methods to assess changes

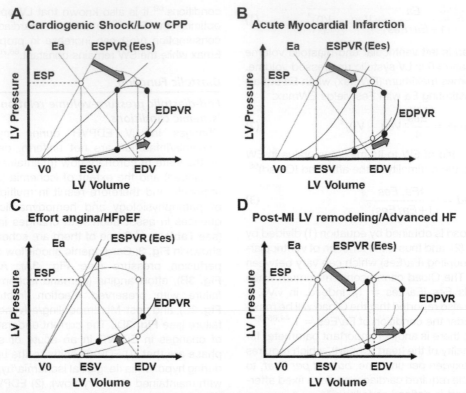

Fig. 3. PV diagram in several cardiac emergencies. (*A*) Cardiogenic shock/low coronary perfusion pressure (CPP): ESPVR slope is reduced, which diminishes stroke volume. (*B*) AMI: ESPVR in bilinear model shifts rightward, which diminishes stroke volume. (*C*) Effort angina (demand ischemia)/heart failure with preserved ejection fraction (HFpEF); EDPVR shifts left upward; and (*D*) Post-myocardial infarction (MI) LV remodeling/advanced heart failure (HF): ESPVR slope is reduced and EDPVR shifts markedly right-downward.

in EDPVR include approximation of EDPVR by a fourth-order polynomial with a dummy variable that quantitatively evaluates an upward shift of EDPVR,[78] and comparisons of LV volumes at a given LVEDP (for example, LVEDV at LVEDP 30 mm Hg) which assesses a rightward or leftward shift of EDPVR.[9]

Left ventricular remodeling

In subacute or chronic phase after AMI, structural changes in LV occur in adaptation to hemodynamic/neurohumoral derangements, including healing and scarring (fibrosis) at the infarct site and mechanical stretch and eccentric hypertrophy at the residual viable myocardium.[79] As a result, the LV diastolic wall stress increases and then the EDPVR can shift rightward toward larger LV volumes.[80] Taken together, these structural and biomechanical alternations are termed as LV remodeling. Factors involved in LV remodeling are shown in **Box 1**. Although not listed in **Box 1**, another potential influencing factor of LV remodeling may be incomplete relaxation. In post-AMI hearts, the rate of LV

relaxation is decreased, and especially at higher heart rates with increased sympathetic nerve activity, incomplete relaxation may occur due to the uncoupling of actin-myosin bonds between contractions.[81] Under these conditions, the LV may not be fully relaxed at end-diastole and result in elevation of LVEDP and diastolic wall stress, thereby contributing to LV remodeling.

Therapies to prevent LV remodeling after AMI include minimizing the infarct size, improving scar formation, diminishing or avoiding infarct expansion, and reducing LV wall stress. LV mechanical unloading is a powerful therapeutic modality to reduce oxygen demand and limit infarct area. Previous studies reported that LV remodeling was reversed with LV assist devices in patients with dilated or ischemic cardiomyopathy.[9] During the acute phase of AMI, LV mechanical unloading with Impella can reduce infarct size and prevent subsequent heart failure by preserving LV systolic function.[82,83] Although further clinical studies are required, the mechanical LV unloading

---

Box 1
Factors involved in left ventricular remodeling

1. Size and site of myocardial infarction

   a. ST elevation due to transmural myocardial infarction

   b. Infarction in anterior wall

   c. Viability of infarct zone

2. Process of treatment

   a. Coronary artery patency of culprit lesion

   b. Collateral flow from other coronary arteries

3. Left ventricular wall stress

   a. Hypertension

   b. Excessive exercise stress

4. Neurohormonal factors

   a. Sympathetic nerve activity

   b. Renin-angiotensin-aldosterone system

   c. Bradykinin

   d. Medication   (angiotensin-converting enzyme inhibitor, angiotensin II receptor blocker, beta-blocker)

---

to diminish the LV wall stress and LV remodeling in the acute phase of AMI is theoretically rational from the point of view of cardiac mechanoenergetics.

Because LV remodeling is an important determinant of long-term prognosis in patients after AMI, it is now a general consensus that patients who are post-AMI should be treated with standard medical therapy with neurohormonal blockers to prevent LV remodeling.[84] The overall mechanisms leading to LV remodeling and heart failure after AMI are complex, including structural, hemodynamic, and neurohormonal processes that result in decreased LV pump performance and impaired peripheral vascular functions.[85]

Cardiac Mechanoenergetics Viewed from Myocardial Oxygen Consumption Pressure-Volume Area Diagram

Left ventricular global function and energetics
Pressure-Volume area as a load-independent determinant of cardiac oxygen consumption In a stable contractility state, Vo_2 linearly correlates with PVA, regardless of mode of contraction (ie, isovolumic or ejecting contraction) under various LV preload and afterload conditions.[48] Because

the experimentally observed Vo_2-PVA relation was highly linear with a correlation coefficient very close to unity (r = 0.96 on average), the following equation was obtained: Vo_2 = a x PVA + b, where a is the slope of the VO_2-PVA relation and b is the Vo_2 intercept (**Fig. 4**A). A correlation coefficient of 0.96 yields a coefficient of determination of 0.92, indicating that approximately 92% of the variance of Vo_2 can be explained by the variance of PVA. Thus, PVA is a load-independent, powerful determinant of Vo_2 under a given stable contractility state.

Total Vo_2 per beat can be divided into PVA-dependent Vo_2 (total mechanical energy) and PVA-independent Vo_2 (VO_2-axis intercept in **Fig. 4**A), which is the sum of excitation-contraction (E-C) coupling and basal metabolism.[48] The slope of the VO_2-PVA relation indicates oxygen cost of PVA or cost of LV mechanical energy.[12] Because the dimensions of both Vo_2 and PVA can be converted to those of energy (J) according to the equations, "1 mL O_2 = 20 J" and "1 mm $Hg \cdot mL$ = 1.33×10^{-4} J," the reciprocal of the slope of the VO_2-PVA relation represents the chemomechanical energy conversion efficiency (ie, contractile efficiency) from Vo_2 used for mechanical contraction (chemical energy) to PVA (total mechanical energy), and the steeper the slope, the less efficient the oxygen cost of mechanical contraction. The contractile efficiency is thought to be the product of conversion efficacy: (1) from PVA-dependent Vo_2 to ATP provided by mitochondrial oxidative phosphorylation, and (2) from the provided ATP to PVA for the contractile machinery. Conversely, the VO_2-axis intercept at zero PVA, that is, PVA-independent Vo_2, reflects Vo_2 used for nonmechanical activities such as Ca^{2+} handling for E-C coupling and basal metabolism to maintain myocardial availability and integrity.[12,48]

Effect of inotropic drugs The VO_2-PVA relation shifts upward parallel with incremental Ees by most positive inotropic drugs, including catecholamines, digitalis, and Ca^{2+}, with an increase in PVA-independent Vo_2 used for E-C coupling[22,48] (**Fig. 4**B). In contrast, negative inotropic agents such as β-blockers, Ca blockers, or fentanyl shift the relation downward parallel with a decrease in PVA-independent Vo_2 (**Fig. 4**C).

In these inotropic interventions, the increase in PVA-independent Vo_2 positively correlates with the increase in contractility (Ees). When increases in PVA-independent Vo_2 at multiple inotropic states are plotted against the corresponding increases in Ees, a linear relation is obtained: PVA-independent Vo_2 = c * Ees + d, where c

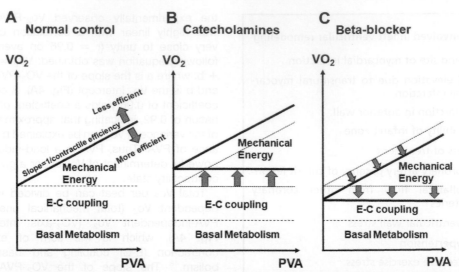

Fig. 4. Schematic diagram of Vo$_2$-PVA relations. (*A*) Normal control: A linear Vo$_2$-PVA relation (*diagonal solid line*) was obtained by changing LV preload and afterload conditions in a stable contractility state. The area under the Vo$_2$-PVA relation is composed of basal metabolism, excitation-contraction coupling (E-C coupling), and mechanical energy (PVA-dependent Vo$_2$). The slope of the diagonal solid line represents an inverse relationship of contractile efficiency (1/contractile efficiency). (*B*) *Catecholamines*: The slope will shift upward parallelly due to increase E-C coupling. Both mechanical energy and basal metabolism are not changed. (*C*) Beta-blocker: E-C coupling will be reduced by beta-blocker. The slope will shift downward parallelly due to decreased E-C coupling.

represents the slope of this relation and d is the PVA-independent Vo$_2$ intercept at zero Ees. The slope c describes "the oxygen cost of contractility," which indicates the increment in Vo$_2$ per unit increment in Ees, reflecting the energy cost for calcium cycling. The oxygen cost of contractility has been reported to be similar between epinephrine and calcium.[48] In contrast, in postreperfusion stunned myocardium, the oxygen cost of contractility has been reported to be increased,[52] suggesting an increased energy cost for calcium cycling. Development of a new inotropic drug with a lower oxygen cost of contractility may be beneficial for patients with heart failure.

Impact of global ischemia (lowering of coronary perfusion pressure) on VO$_2$-PVA relation Suga and colleagues[54] studied the effect of decreased coronary perfusion pressure on the VO$_2$-PVA relation. In excised cross-circulated dog hearts, a decrease in coronary perfusion pressure (from 82 to 51 mm Hg) diminished Ees by 17% and slight decrease in VO$_2$-PVA relationship in a parallel fashion. A further decrease in coronary perfusion pressure (to 32 mm Hg) led to a decrease in Ees by 56% and considerably depressed the VO$_2$-PVA relationship by decreasing both the VO$_2$-axis intercept and the slope of Ees. These results might be superficially interpreted as such that LV contractile efficiency is increased (ie, oxygen

cost of PVA is decreased) despite lowering coronary perfusion pressure. However, the correct interpretation should be that, as PVA is progressively increased, Ees and hence PVA-independent Vo$_2$ progressively decrease due to an excessive LV load, forming a new VO2-PVA relation downward (**Fig. 5**). Thus the newly synthesized composite VO$_2$-PVA relation has a seemingly lower slope value, which might have been erroneously interpreted as an improved contractile efficiency.

Regional myocardial function and energetics
Regional work Because LV myocardial function is impaired nonuniformly in patients with AMI and because global indexes of LV function such as LV ejection fraction cannot detect regional abnormalities of myocardial contractile function, diagnosis and treatment of these patients should be based on correct assessment of LV regional contractile function (**Fig. 6**). To quantify regional contractile function, many variables have been proposed (**Box 2**), and among these, the amount of myocardial shortening, wall thickening, or the regional work index have been conventionally used.[19] However, the relation between these variables and regional myocardial Vo$_2$ under various conditions has not been fully investigated, and more importantly, none of these variables have dimensions of energy that are generated by contraction of the LV region.

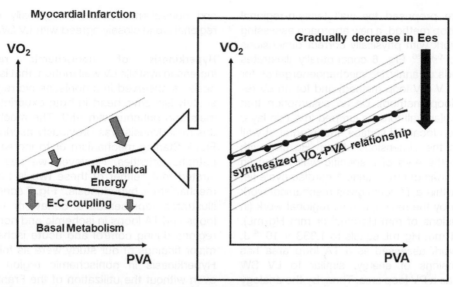

Fig. 5. Mechanism of decreased slope of Vo_2-PVA relationship under lowering coronary perfusion pressure. As PVA increases, Ees decreases under lower coronary perfusion pressure. This newly synthesized Vo_2-PVA relationship has a lower slope, which reflects decreased efficiency.

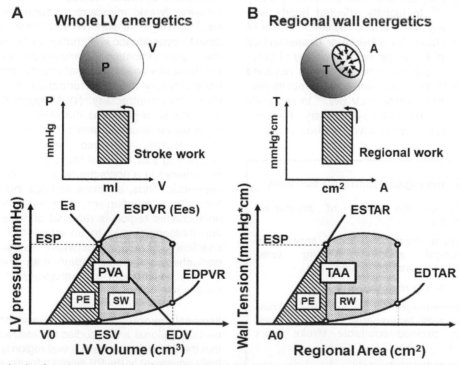

Fig. 6. Methods of analyzing LV global (A) and regional (B) mechanics and energetics using PV loops and wall TA loops. EW performed by the whole LV and by a region on the LV surface can be assessed from the areas within the PV and TA loops, respectively. The total mechanical energy expenditure is represented by systolic PVA for the whole LV and TAA for the region. Both PVA and TAA consist of 2 portions of PE and EW (SW and RW, respectively), and have the dimensions of energy because 1 mm Hg·cm^3 = 1.33 × 10^{-4} J. A, area; A0, unstressed area; P, pressure; RW, regional work; T, tension; V, volume; V0, unstressed LV volume.

We have proposed the wall tension-regional area (TA) loop method, a new approach assessing regional work with physically correct dimensions of energy.[1,6,19,86] **Fig. 6** conceptually illustrates the methods of analyzing mechanoenergetics for the whole LV (PV loop method) and for an LV region (TA loop method). On an assumption that the ventricular wall force is lumped in a thin layer of the LV endocardial surface, the integral of wall tension (in the dimensions of mm Hg·cm) with respect to the area of a specific wall region (in the dimensions of cm^2) during 1 cardiac cycle (ie, the area within a TA loop) gives mechanical work performed by the region, that is, regional work (in the dimensions of mm Hg·cm,[3] or mm Hg·mL). Because 1 mm Hg·mL equals to 1.333×10^{-4} J, regional work assessed as a TA loop area has the dimensions of energy, similar to LV SW assessed as a PV loop area. Then, by the analogy of LV PV diagram, one can derive end-systolic TA relation (ESTAR), end-diastolic TA relation (EDTAR), and systolic TA area (TAA) (see **Fig. 6**).

The TA loop method for the assessment of regional work has been experimentally validated under 2 situations: (1) globally affected hearts (alterations of LV loading conditions and contractility), and (2) regionally ischemic hearts (coronary artery obstruction).[6,86] In globally affected hearts with altered stroke volume or end-diastolic volume at enhanced (dobutamine infusion) or depressed LV contractility (global ischemia by lowering of coronary perfusion pressure), regional work obtained from the TA loop method well agreed with its predicted value obtained from LV SW.[86] In regionally ischemic hearts produced by coronary artery occlusion, the sum of regional work for both ischemic and nonischemic zones (ie, globally integrated regional work) closely agreed with LV SW.[6]

Hyperkinesis of nonischemic regions An increased systolic LV wall motion, that is, hyperkinesis, is observed in a nonischemic region of an acutely ischemic heart in both experimental animals and patients with AMI. The mechanism of this hyperkinesis was previously ascribed to the Frank-Starling mechanism or to increased sympathetic activities. However, we have demonstrated that neither of these two is the primary mechanism of hyperkinesis.[1] **Fig. 7** schematically illustrates representative behaviors of LV PV loops and TA loops in ischemic and nonischemic regions during control and acute ischemia. The major findings of our study were as follows.[1] (1) Hyperkinesis in nonischemic region occurred even without the utilization of the Frank-Starling mechanism in an isolated heart with LV end-diastolic and stroke volumes kept constant. (2) Area shrinkage and reciprocal area expansion in an isovolumic contraction period occurred concomitantly in nonischemic and ischemic regions, respectively, during acute ischemia, indicating an intraventricular regional mechanical interaction between nonischemic (strong) and ischemic (weak) myocardium connected in series.[87] (3) Regional work (TA loop area) decreased despite hyperkinetic wall motion in the nonischemic region, indicating hyperkinesis is ascribed to mechanical unloading of that region rather than a compensatory hyper-performance or enhanced myocardial contractility. (4) Although ESTAR in an ischemic region was markedly shifted rightward during acute ischemia, that in a nonischemic region remained almost constant, suggesting that regional myocardial contractility is unaltered in a nonischemic region despite hyperkinesis. Thus, all these findings indicate that the primary mechanism of hyperkinesis in the nonischemic region is regional afterload reduction (unloading) due to an intraventricular mechanical interaction between ischemic and nonischemic regions rather than the Frank-Starling mechanism or enhanced myocardial contractility.[1]

Regional myocardial oxygen consumption and tension-regional area Studies to date have shown that the TA diagram for an LV wall region is energetically equivalent to the PV diagram for the whole LV. Then, by the analogy of LV PVA, systolic TAA in the TA diagram is considered to represent regional total mechanical energy generated by the regional myocardial contraction (see **Fig. 6**). To test this hypothesis, correlations between regional Vo_2 and 3

Box 2
Indexes of the regional contractile functions

1. Indexes of the extent of myocardial shortening

   Segment shortening, chord shortening, fractional area, shortening (area shrinkage), wall thickening

2. Indexes of the regional work

   Pressure-length loop, pressure-thickness loop, wall tension-area loop, wall-stress loop, preload-recruitable stroke work index

3. Indexes as the end-systole

   End-systolic pressure-length relation, end-systolic pressure-thickness relation, end-systolic tension-area relation, end-systolic stress relation

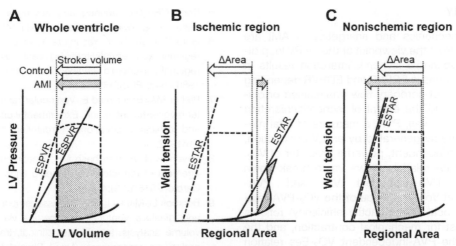

Fig. 7. Schematic illustration of representative behaviors of PV loops and TA loops before and during acute ischemia. LV PV loops (*A*) and TA loops in ischemic (*B*) and nonischemic regions (*C*) before (Control) and during acute ischemia at constant LV end-diastolic and end-systolic volumes are shown. It is of note that, during regional ischemia, the slope of the ESPVR decreased and ESTAR of the ischemic region markedly shifts rightward, whereas ESTAR of the nonischemic region remains almost constant. Arrows indicate stroke volume and the amount of regional area shrinkage (ΔArea) during the control period (*open arrows*) and regional ischemia (*shaded arrows*).

variables of regional mechanical performance (ie, regional area shrinkage, regional work, and TAA) were examined under various LV preload, afterload, and contraction modes (isovolumic vs ejecting contractions).[19] The results indicated that only TAA correlates with regional Vo_2 in a highly linear manner regardless of LV loading conditions (**Fig. 8**). Thus, TAA is a powerful mechanical predictor of regional Vo_2.

Interestingly, the slope of the regional Vo_2-TAA relationship was remarkably consistent among the different hearts or different LV preload and afterload conditions and close to the reported value for the slope of LV Vo_2-PVA relation.[19] Because the reciprocal of the LV Vo_2-PVA relation indicates contractile efficiency, which is a chemomechanical energy conversion efficiency from oxygen used exclusively for mechanical contraction to total mechanical energy generated by a contraction,[23,48] the close agreement between the slopes of regional Vo_2-TAA and LV Vo_2-PVA relations also supports the validity of TAA as a measure of regional mechanical energy expenditure. Thus, TAA is a powerful tool to investigate the relation between regional mechanics and energetics in the LV.

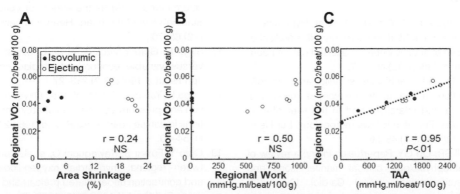

Fig. 8. Examples of correlations between regional Vo_2 and variables of regional mechanical performance in a representative heart. Among the 3 variables of regional mechanical performance, only TAA (Panel C) highly linearly correlates with regional Vo_2 regardless of contraction mode or loading conditions, whereas area shrinkage (Panel A) and regional work (Panel B) do not.

SUMMARY

Cardiac mechanics and energetics in AMI are described from the viewpoint of the LV PV loop diagram. Myocardial ischemia/infarction results in various changes in ESPVR and EDPVR depending on the state of coronary flow (maintained or discontinued) and the extent of ischemia/infarction (global or regional), PVA, a measure of total mechanical energy generated by an LV contraction, is a load-independent, powerful predictor of Vo_2. The VO_2-PVA relation allows us to break down Vo_2 into PVA-dependent Vo_2 and PVA-independent Vo_2. The slope of the VO_2-PVA relation (reciprocal of contractile efficiency) reflects energy cost for mechanical contraction, and the slope of the PVA-independent VO_2-Ees relation (oxygen cost of contractility) reflects energy cost for E-C coupling. Finally, by the analogy of the global PV diagram, regional TA diagram gives regional work (TA loop area), regional myocardial contractility (ESTAR), and regional energetics (regional VO_2-TAA relation). Taken together, these new frameworks may help us to understand pathophysiology and to develop a new treatment strategy in patients with AMI and/or heart failure.

ACKNOWLEDGMENTS

We appreciate Rakushumimarika Harada and Yogamaya Mantha for editing the article.

CONFLICT OF INTEREST

None.

DISCLOSURE

The authors have nothing to disclose.

REFERENCES

1. Goto Y, Igarashi Y, Yamada O, et al. Hyperkinesis without the Frank-Starling mechanism in a nonischemic region of acutely ischemic excised canine heart. Circulation 1988;77(2):468–77.
2. Swan HJ. Left ventricular systolic and diastolic dysfunction in the acute phases of myocardial ischaemia and infarction, and in the later phases of recovery. Function follows morphology. Eur Heart J 1993;14(Suppl A):48–56.
3. Maxwell SR, Lip GY. Reperfusion injury: a review of the pathophysiology, clinical manifestations and therapeutic options. Int J Cardiol 1997;58(2): 95–117.
4. Guaricci AI, Bulzis G, Pontone G, et al. Current interpretation of myocardial stunning. Trends Cardiovasc Med 2018;28(4):263–71.
5. Conti CR. The stunned and hibernating myocardium: a brief review. Clin Cardiol 1991;14(9):708–12.
6. Goto Y, Igarashi Y, Yasumura Y, et al. Integrated regional work equals total left ventricular work in regionally ischemic canine heart. Am J Physiol 1988;254(5 Pt 2):H894–904.
7. Pfeffer MA, Braunwald E. Ventricular remodeling after myocardial infarction. Experimental observations and clinical implications. Circulation 1990;81(4): 1161–72.
8. Reyentovich A, Barghash MH, Hochman JS. Management of refractory cardiogenic shock. Nat Rev Cardiol 2016;13(8):481–92.
9. Burkhoff D, Mirsky I, Suga H. Assessment of systolic and diastolic ventricular properties via pressure-volume analysis: a guide for clinical, translational, and basic researchers. Am J Physiol Heart Circ Physiol 2005;289(2):H501–12.
10. Suga H, Sagawa K. Graphical estimation of ventricular wall force and stress from pressure-volume diagram. Am J Physiol 1979;236(6):H787–9.
11. Suga H. Cardiac energetics: from E(max) to pressure-volume area. Clin Exp Pharmacol Physiol 2003;30(8):580–5.
12. Suga H. Paul Dudley White International Lecture: cardiac performance as viewed through the pressure-volume window. Jpn Heart J 1994;35(3): 263–80.
13. Khalafbeigui F, Suga H, Sagawa K. Left ventricular systolic pressure-volume area correlates with oxygen consumption. Am J Physiol 1979;237(5): H566–9.
14. Suga H, Goto Y, Yamada O, et al. Independence of myocardial oxygen consumption from pressure-volume trajectory during diastole in canine left ventricle. Circ Res 1984;55(6):734–9.
15. Suga H. Total mechanical energy of a ventricle model and cardiac oxygen consumption. Am J Physiol 1979;236(3):H498–505.
16. Suga H, Goto Y, Futaki S, et al. Systolic pressure-volume area (PVA) as the energy of contraction in Starling's law of the heart. Heart and vessels 1991; 6(2):65–70.
17. Suga H, Goto Y, Hata K, et al. Constant efficiency versus variable economy of cardiac contraction. Jpn Heart J 1992;33(2):213–27.
18. Suga H, Yamada O, Goto Y, et al. Oxygen consumption and pressure-volume area of abnormal contractions in canine heart. Am J Physiol 1984;246(2 Pt 2): H154–60.
19. Goto Y, Futaki S, Kawaguchi O, et al. Coupling between regional myocardial oxygen consumption and contraction under altered preload and afterload. J Am Coll Cardiol 1993;21(6):1522–31.
20. Green P, Kodali S, Leon MB, et al. Echocardiographic assessment of pressure volume relations in heart failure and valvular heart disease: using

imaging to understand physiology. Minerva Cardi-oangiol 2011;59(4):375–89.

21. de Simone G, Izzo R, Losi MA, et al. Depressed myocardial energetic efficiency is associated with increased cardiovascular risk in hypertensive left ventricular hypertrophy. J Hypertens 2016;34(9): 1846–53.

22. Suga H, Hisano R, Goto Y, et al. Effect of positive inotropic agents on the relation between oxygen consumption and systolic pressure volume area in canine left ventricle. Circ Res 1983;53(3): 306–18.

23. Suga H, Yamada O, Goto Y, et al. Constant me-chanical efficiency of contractile machinery of canine left ventricle under different loading and inotropic conditions. Jpn J Physiol 1984;34(4): 679–98.

24. Ohgoshi Y, Goto Y, Futaki S, et al. Sensitivities of car-diac O2 consumption and contractility to catechol-amines in dogs. Am J Physiol 1991;261(1 Pt 2): H196–205.

25. Suga H, Yamada O, Goto Y. Energetics of ventricular contraction as traced in the pressure-volume dia-gram. Fed Proc 1984;43(9):2411–3.

26. Hata K, Goto Y, Futaki S, et al. Mechanoenergetic ef-fects of pimobendan in canine left ventricles. Com-parison with dobutamine. Circulation 1992;86(4): 1291–301.

27. Suga H, Sagawa K. Instantaneous pressure-volume relationships and their ratio in the excised, supported canine left ventricle. Circ Res 1974;35(1):117–26.

28. Chen CH, Nakayama M, Nevo E, et al. Coupled systolic-ventricular and vascular stiffening with age: implications for pressure regulation and car-diac reserve in the elderly. J Am Coll Cardiol 1998; 32(5):1221–7.

29. Suga H, Sagawa K, Kostiuk DP. Controls of ventric-ular contractility assessed by pressure-volume ration, Emax. Cardiovasc Res 1976;10(5):582–92.

30. Kono A, Maughan WL, Sunagawa K, et al. The use of left ventricular end-ejection pressure and peak pres-sure in the estimation of the end-systolic pressure-volume relationship. Circulation 1984;70(6): 1057–65.

31. Kass DA, Yamazaki T, Burkhoff D, et al. Determina-tion of left ventricular end-systolic pressure-volume relationships by the conductance (volume) catheter technique. Circulation 1986;73(3):586–95.

32. Suga H, Goto Y, Igarashi Y, et al. Ventricular suction under zero source pressure for filling. Am J Physiol 1986;251(1 Pt 2):H47–55.

33. Suga H, Sagawa K, Shoukas AA. Load independence of the instantaneous pressure-volume ratio of the canine left ventricle and effects of epinephrine and heart rate on the ratio. Circ Res 1973;32(3):314–22.

34. Parmley WW, Tyberg JV, Glantz SA. Cardiac dy-namics. Annu Rev Physiol 1977;39:277–99.

35. Borbely A, van der Velden J, Papp Z, et al. Cardio-myocyte stiffness in diastolic heart failure. Circula-tion 2005;111(6):774–81.

36. Diamond G, Forrester JS, Hargis J, et al. Diastolic pressure-volume relationship in the canine left ventricle. Circ Res 1971;29(3):267–75.

37. Levis BS, Gotsman MS. Current concepts of left ven-tricular relaxation and compliance. Am Heart J 1980; 99:101–12.

38. Labeit S, Kolmerer B. Titins: giant proteins in charge of muscle ultrastructure and elasticity. Science 1995; 270(5234):293–6.

39. LeWinter MM, Granzier H. Cardiac titin: a multifunc-tional giant. Circulation 2010;121(19):2137–45.

40. Zile MR, Baicu CF, Ikonomidis JS, et al. Myocardial stiffness in patients with heart failure and a pre-served ejection fraction: contributions of collagen and titin. Circulation 2015;131(14):1247–59.

41. Zile MR, Baicu CF, Gaasch WH. Diastolic heart fail-ure–abnormalities in active relaxation and passive stiffness of the left ventricle. N Engl J Med 2004; 350(19):1953–9.

42. Hamdani N, Herwig M, Linke WA. Tampering with springs: phosphorylation of titin affecting the me-chanical function of cardiomyocytes. Biophys Rev 2017;9(3):225–37.

43. Sunagawa K, Maughan WL, Burkhoff D, et al. Left ventricular interaction with arterial load studied in isolated canine ventricle. Am J Physiol 1983;245(5 Pt 1):H773–80.

44. Sunagawa K, Maughan WL, Sagawa K. Optimal arterial resistance for the maximal stroke work stud-ied in isolated canine left ventricle. Circ Res 1985; 56(4):586–95.

45. Walley KR. Left ventricular function: time-varying elastance and left ventricular aortic coupling. Crit Care 2016;20:270.

46. Takaoka H, Takeuchi M, Odake M, et al. Comparison of the effects on arterial-ventricular coupling be-tween phosphodiesterase inhibitor and dobutamine in the diseased human heart. J Am Coll Cardiol 1993;22(2):598–606.

47. Chantler PD, Lakatta EG, Najjar SS. Arterial-ventric-ular coupling: mechanistic insights into cardiovascu-lar performance at rest and during exercise. J Appl Physiol 2008;105(4):1342–51.

48. Suga H. Ventricular energetics. Physiol Rev 1990; 70(2):247–77.

49. Kameyama T, Asanoi H, Ishizaka S, et al. Energy conversion efficiency in human left ventricle. Circula-tion 1992;85(3):988–96.

50. Suga H, Tanaka N, Ohgoshi Y, et al. Hyperthyroid dog left ventricle has the same oxygen consumption versus pressure-volume area (PVA) relation as euthyroid dog. Heart Vessels 1991;6(2):71–83.

51. Goto Y, Futaki S, Kawaguchi O, et al. Left ventricular contractility and energetic cost in disease models–

an approach from the pressure-volume diagram. Jpn Circ J 1992;56(7):716–21.

52. Ohgoshi Y, Goto Y, Futaki S, et al. Increased oxygen cost of contractility in stunned myocardium of dogs. Circ Res 1991;69:975–88.

53. Suga H, Yasumura Y, Nozawa T, et al. Prospective prediction of O2 consumption from pressure-volume area in dog hearts. Am J Physiol 1987; 252(6 Pt 2):H1258–64.

54. Suga H, Goto Y, Yasumura Y, et al. O2 consumption of dog heart under decreased coronary perfusion and propranolol. Am J Physiol 1988;254(2 Pt 2): H292–303.

55. Suga H, Goto Y, Nozawa T, et al. Force-time integral decreases with ejection despite constant oxygen consumption and pressure-volume area in dog left ventricle. Circ Res 1987;60(6):797–803.

56. Kawaguchi O, Goto Y, Ohgoshi Y, et al. Dynamic cardiac compression improves contractile efficiency of the heart. J Thorac Cardiovasc Surg 1997;113(5): 923–31.

57. Suga H, Igarashi Y, Yamada O, et al. Mechanical efficiency of the left ventricle as a function of preload, afterload, and contractility. Heart Vessels 1985;1(1):3–8.

58. Schaff HV, Gott VL, Goldman RA, et al. Mechanism of elevated left ventricular end-diastolic pressure after ischemic arrest and reperfusion. Am J Physiol 1981;240(2):H300–7.

59. Palacios I, Johnson RA, Newell JB, et al. Left ventricular end-diastolic pressure volume relationships with experimental acute global ischemia. Circulation 1976;53(3):428–36.

60. Zile MR, Izzi G, Gaasch WH. Left ventricular diastolic dysfunction limits use of maximum systolic elastance as an index of contractile function. Circulation 1991;83(2):674–80.

61. Sunagawa K, Maughan WL, Friesinger G, et al. Effects of coronary arterial pressure on left ventricular end-systolic pressure-volume relation of isolated canine heart. Circ Res 1982;50(5):727–34.

62. Sunagawa K, Maughan WL, Sagawa K. Effect of regional ischemia on the left ventricular end-systolic pressure-volume relationship of isolated canine hearts. Circ Res 1983;52(2):170–8.

63. Kass DA, Marino P, Maughan WL, et al. Determinants of end-systolic pressure-volume relations during acute regional ischemia in situ. Circulation 1989; 80(6):1783–94.

64. Burkhoff D, Sugiura S, Yue DT, et al. Contractility-dependent curvilinearity of end-systolic pressure-volume relations. Am J Physiol 1987;252(6 Pt 2): H1218–27.

65. Burkhoff D, Sagawa K. Ventricular efficiency predicted by an analytical model. Am J Physiol 1986; 250(6 Pt 2):R1021–7.

66. Kubota T, Alexander J Jr, Itaya R, et al. Dynamic effects of carotid sinus baroreflex on ventriculoarterial coupling studied in anesthetized dogs. Circ Res 1992;70(5):1044–53.

67. Hata K, Goto Y, Suga H. External mechanical work during relaxation period does not affect myocardial oxygen consumption. Am J Physiol 1991;261(6 Pt 2):H1778–84.

68. Sunagawa K, Sugimachi M, Todaka K, et al. Optimal coupling of the left ventricle with the arterial system. Basic Res Cardiol 1993;88(Suppl 2):75–90.

69. De Tombe PP, Jones S, Burkhoff D, et al. Ventricular stroke work and efficiency both remain nearly optimal despite altered vascular loading. Am J Physiol 1993;264(6 Pt 2):H1817–24.

70. Tanaka N, Nozawa T, Yasumura Y, et al. Contractility to minimize oxygen consumption for constant work in dog left ventricle. Heart Vessels 1990; 6(1):9–20.

71. Sugimachi M, Todaka K, Sunagawa K, et al. Optimal afterload for the heart vs. optimal heart for the afterload. Front Med Biol Eng 1990;2(3):217–21.

72. Goto Y. Ischemic myocardium: mechanical property of ischemic myocardium. Nihon Rinsho 2003;61(4): 107–12 [in Japanese].

73. Wyman RM, Farhi ER, Bing OH, et al. Comparative effects of hypoxia and ischemia in the isolated, blood-perfused dog heart: evaluation of left ventricular diastolic chamber distensibility and wall thickness. Circ Res 1989;64(1):121–8.

74. Visner MS, Arentzen CE, Parrish DG, et al. Effects of global ischemia on the diastolic properties of the left ventricle in the conscious dog. Circulation 1985; 71(3):610–9.

75. Mann T, Brodie BR, Grossman W, et al. Effect of angina on the left ventricular diastolic pressure-volume relationship. Circulation 1977;55(5): 761–6.

76. Goto Y. Pathophysiology of diastolic heart failure: understanding physiological pathologies. Respir Circ 2009;57(3):245–55 [in Japanese].

77. Glantz SA. Computing indices of diastolic stiffness has been counterproductive. Fed Proc 1980;39(2): 162–8.

78. Goto Y, Yamamoto J, Saito M, et al. Effects of right ventricular ischemia on left ventricular geometry and the end-diastolic pressure-volume relationship in the dog. Circulation 1985;72(5):1104–14.

79. Anversa P, Olivetti G, Capasso JM. Cellular basis of ventricular remodeling after myocardial infarction. Am J Cardiol 1991;68(14):7d–16d.

80. Uriel N, Sayer G, Annamalai S, et al. Mechanical unloading in heart failure. J Am Coll Cardiol 2018; 72(5):569–80.

81. Runte KE, Bell SP, Selby DE, et al. Relaxation and the role of calcium in isolated contracting myocardium from patients with hypertensive heart

disease and heart failure with preserved ejection fraction. Circ Heart Fail 2017;10(8) [pii: e004311].

82. Saku K, Kakino T, Arimura T, et al. Left ventricular mechanical unloading by total support of impella in myocardial infarction reduces infarct size, preserves left ventricular function, and prevents subsequent heart failure in dogs. Circ Heart Fail 2018;11(5): e004397.

83. Kapur NK, Paruchuri V, Urbano-Morales JA, et al. Mechanically unloading the left ventricle before coronary reperfusion reduces left ventricular wall stress and myocardial infarct size. Circulation 2013;128(4): 328–36.

84. Angeli FS, Shapiro M, Amabile N, et al. Left ventricular remodeling after myocardial infarction: characterization of a swine model on beta-blocker therapy. Comp Med 2009;59(3):272–9.

85. Francis GS. Pathophysiology of chronic heart failure. Am J Med 2001;110(Suppl 7A):37s–46s.

86. Goto Y, Suga H, Yamada O, et al. Left ventricular regional work from wall tension-area loop in canine heart. Am J Physiol 1986;250:H151–8.

87. Wiegner AW, Allen GJ, Bing OH. Weak and strong myocardium in series: implications for segmental dysfunction. Am J Physiol 1978;235: H776–83.

Noninvasive Positive Pressure Ventilation for Acute Decompensated Heart Failure

Michinari Hieda, MD, MSc, PhD[a,b]

KEYWORDS

- Acute decompensated heart failure • Cardiogenic pulmonary edema
- Noninvasive positive pressure ventilation (NIPPV) • Positive airway pressure (PAP)
- Bilevel positive airway pressure (Bilevel PAP) • Adaptive servoventilation (ASV)
- Transmural pressure

KEY POINTS

- Noninvasive positive pressure ventilation (NIPPV) devices, including continuous positive airway pressure (PAP), bilevel PAP, and adaptive servoventilation, are noninvasive therapeutic tools for patients with acute decompensated heart failure and cardiogenic pulmonary edema.
- PAP therapy can provide favorable effects on not only lung functions and pulmonary circulation but also systemic hemodynamics, which can reduce the intubation rate and improve clinical symptoms and mortality in patients with cardiogenic pulmonary edema.
- PAP devices have a favorable potential to improve oxygenation, and to provide pulmonary recruitment, increased functional residual lung capacity, and decreased right ventricular (RV) preload and afterload, diminished left ventricular (LV) afterload, eventually to stabilize hemodynamics.
- The hemodynamic net effect of positive end-expiratory pressure on cardiac output depends on both RV and LV functions, LV preload, and LV afterload; therefore, the elucidating hemodynamics and cardiac functions are paramount.

INTRODUCTION

Despite the establishment of standard therapy for heart failure, it still remains a devastating disease that affects 6.5 million Americans ≥20 years of age.[1] The prevalence of heart failure has exponentially increased 46% from 2012 to 2030 in the United States.[2] The prognosis of heart failure is worsening over time, and especially advanced heart failure is associated with dramatic reductions in quality of life and high mortality and comorbidity.[3–6] As the severity of heart failure increases, the intensity of care will escalate in parallel, and then the recovery from heart failure exacerbations will be difficult, which gradually and eventually leads to death.[7] Therefore, an appropriate early therapeutic intervention becomes paramount in achieving patient recovery.

In 1936, Poulton[8] reported for the first time that "pulmonary plus pressure machine" provided by an Electrolux or Hoover vacuum cleaner was a useful therapeutic tool for patients with acute

Funding: Dr M. Hieda was supported in part by the American Heart Association Strategically Focused Research Network (14SFRN20600009-03). Dr M. Hieda was also supported by American Heart Association postdoctoral fellowship grant (18POST33960092) and the Harry S. Moss Heart Trust.
a University of Texas Southwestern Medical Center, Institute for Exercise and Environmental Medicine, Texas Health Presbyterian Hospital, 7232 Greenville Avenue, Dallas, TX 75231, USA; b Kyushu University, School of Medicine, Department of Medicine and Biosystemic Science, Division of Cardiology, 3-1-1 Maidashi Higashi-ku Fukuoka City, Clinical Research Building B6F Fukuoka, Zip:812-8582, Japan
E-mail addresses: hieda.michinari.0119@gmail.com; hieda-m@med.kyushu-u.ac.jp

Heart Failure Clin 16 (2020) 271–282
https://doi.org/10.1016/j.hfc.2020.02.005
1551-7136/20/© 2020 Elsevier Inc. All rights reserved.

cardiogenic pulmonary edema. Since then, technology and noninvasive positive pressure ventilation (NIPPV) have become much more sophisticated.[9] In the emergency room or intensive care unit, NIPPV, providing positive airway pressure (PAP), has been widely used in the management of patients with cardiogenic pulmonary edema.[10–19] The PAP devices, which can be applied without endotracheal airway or tracheostomy, include continuous positive airway pressure (CPAP), bilevel PAP, and adaptive servoventilation (ASV).[20,21] The physiologic effects of PAP consist of improved oxygenation and respiratory mechanics, reduced systemic venous return (VR) resulting in decrease preload of the right ventricle (RV), decreased RV and left ventricular (LV) afterload because of decreased transmural pressure, and reduced excessive sympathetic nerve activity,[22,23] which eventually augments cardiac output. The aim of this review is to explain and evaluate (1) the pathophysiology of acute pulmonary edema, (2) the effects of PAP on physiologic effects and hemodynamics, and (3) the evidence of NIPPV for patients with acute decompensated heart failure (ADHF).

PATHOPHYSIOLOGY OF CARDIOGENIC PULMONARY EDEMA IN ACUTE DECOMPENSATED HEART FAILURE

ADHF is defined as a rapid worsening change in heart failure signs and symptoms,[24,25] such as an aggressive dyspnea with air hunger, productive cough, and pulmonary edema.[3,26,27] Cardiogenic pulmonary edema causing severe respiratory distress with oxygen less than 90% is the most common presentation, and it is a life-threatening emergency.[3,26–28] It is characterized by excessive pulmonary extravascular fluid, which can cause a decrease in lung compliance and diffusing capacity, arterial hypoxemia resulting in increased pulmonary vascular resistance (PVR), airway resistance, and retention of CO_2.[29–31]

The fluid in the interstitial space will move outward from the pulmonary capillary to the interstitial space following the net balance between hydrostatic pressure and plasma protein osmotic pressure,[32] the so-called Starling equation (**Fig. 1**). In the normal, healthy lung, the fluid is leaked through small gaps between pulmonary capillary endothelial cells. Almost all of the excessive unnecessary fluid will be removed by the lymphatics, and it will return to the systemic circulation.[32,33]

On the other hand, in cardiogenic pulmonary edema, the net transvascular flow balance is disrupted because of the rapidly increasing hydrostatic pressure in the capillary owing to increased pulmonary venous pressure from elevated left ventricular end-diastolic pressure (LVEDP).[30,33] The increased hydrostatic pressure in the capillary will provide increased fluid filtration, which is the one of the hallmarks of cardiogenic pulmonary edema (**Table 1**).[34] The elevation of left atrial pressure (LAP) ≥ 18 mm Hg can provide pulmonary edematous change in the peribronchovascular interstitial space.[32] When the LAP increases ≥ 25 mm Hg, the edema fluid breaks through the pulmonary capillary epithelium, resulting in flash pulmonary edema.[32] The liquid-filled alveoli leads to alveolar shrinkage, which provides impaired venous admixture and arterial hypoxemia, resulting in increased PVR.[35,36] Both the liquid-filled alveoli and the higher PVR will be a trigger to the vicious cycle of the cardiogenic pulmonary edema.

EFFECTS OF POSITIVE AIRWAY PRESSURE ON PHYSIOLOGIC EFFECTS AND HEMODYNAMICS

Hemodynamic net effect of positive end-expiratory pressure (PEEP) on cardiac output depends on both RV and LV functions, preload, and afterload.[37] PAP reduces VR and RV preload,[38] but the response afterward depends on the afterload-dependent and the preload-dependent state.[10] Therefore, evaluation of the hemodynamics and cardiac functions is very important.[39]

In Predominantly Afterload-Dependent State (= More Sensitive to Left Ventricular Afterload, eg, Heart Failure with Reduced Ejection Fraction)

PAP decreases VR and RV preload by elevating intrathoracic pressure.[40] The reduction of RV preload can normalize the dilated RV with ventricular septal shift toward the LV, which enables RV/LV to regain shape and wall motion.[41] In addition, PAP can also improve gas exchange and oxygenation through alveoli recruitment, which will attenuate the elevated PVR because of hypoxic pulmonary vasoconstriction and RV-PA (pulmonary artery) coupling.[42] PAP also can decrease LV transmural pressure and increase pressure gradient between the intrathoracic aorta and the extrathoracic systemic circuit, resulting in reduced LV afterload. Reducing sympathetic nerve activity provided by PAP also may contribute to decreasing both RV and LV afterload. The net balance, among reduction in RV preload, greater decrease in PVR, normalizing RV/LV shape, and reduced LV afterload, will lead to improved stroke volume and cardiac output (**Fig. 2**A).[43]

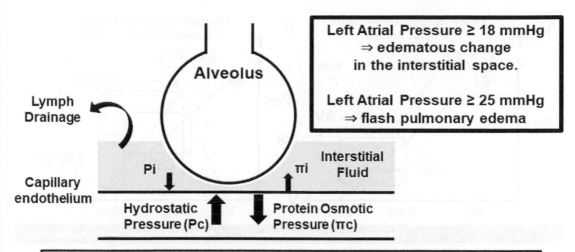

Fig. 1. Physiology of the fluid in the peribronchovascular interstitial space. In the normal, healthy lung, the fluid in peribronchovascular interstitial space is removed by the lymph drainage, and it is returned to the systemic circulation. On In the other hand, in the lung in patients with advanced decompensated heart failure or cardiogenic pulmonary edema, the hydrostatic pressure is increased because of increased LV end-diastolic pressure because of LV systolic and/or diastolic dysfunction, which leads to the increased transvascular fluid filtration.

Table 1
Chest radiographic and echocardiographic characteristics cardiogenic pulmonary edema versus noncardiogenic edema

Radiographic Characteristics	Cardiogenic Pulmonary Edema	Noncardiogenic Edema
Cardiac silhouette	Enlarged	Normal
Distribution of edema	Central infiltrates	Peripheral or patchy infiltrates
Septal lines	Present	Not usually
Peribronchial cuffing	Present (S6)	Not usually
Kerley B lines	Present	Not usually
Pleural effusions	Present	Not usually
Air bronchograms	Not usually	Present
Echocardiographic Characteristics	**Cardiogenic Pulmonary Edema**	**Noncardiogenic Edema**
Pleural effusions	Occasionally present	Not usually, but possible
Ultrasound comet-tail images	Possible present	Not usually

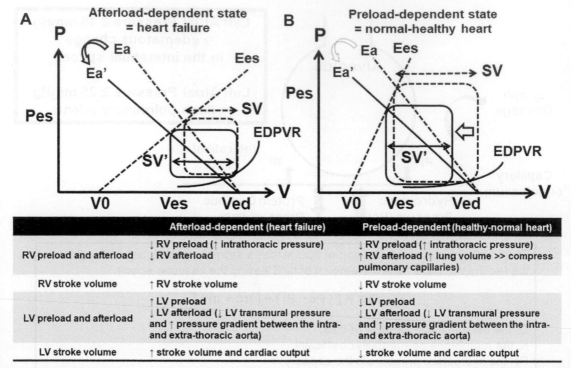

	Afterload-dependent (heart failure)	Preload-dependent (healthy-normal heart)
RV preload and afterload	↓ RV preload (↑ intrathoracic pressure) ↓ RV afterload	↓ RV preload (↑ intrathoracic pressure) ↑ RV afterload (↑ lung volume >> compress pulmonary capillaries)
RV stroke volume	↑ RV stroke volume	↓ RV stroke volume
LV preload and afterload	↑ LV preload ↓ LV afterload (↓ LV transmural pressure and ↑ pressure gradient between the intra- and extra-thoracic aorta)	↓ LV preload ↓ LV afterload (↓ LV transmural pressure and ↑ pressure gradient between the intra- and extra-thoracic aorta)
LV stroke volume	↑ stroke volume and cardiac output	↓ stroke volume and cardiac output

Fig. 2. LV pressure-volume loop showing the effects of PAP on stroke volume in the afterload-dependent (*A*) state versus the preload-dependent state (*B*). The Ees and EDPVR in the afterload-dependent state is less steep and steeper than those in the preload-dependent state. Assuming that Ea has decreased equally by PAP treatment (*from broken line to solid line by PAP treatment*), the stroke volume in the afterload-dependent state will be increased (*A*), but decreased in the preload-dependent state (*B*). Owing to the difference in the response of RV afterload, whereas PAP can improve stroke volume in the afterload-dependent state, PAP may decrease stroke volume in the preload-dependent state, oppositely. Ea, effective arterial elastance; EDPVR, end-diastolic pressure-volume relationship; Ees, end-systolic elastance; P, pressure of the left ventricle; Pes, left ventricular pressure at end-systole; SV, stroke volume; SV', changed stroke volume by PAP treatment; V, volume of the left ventricle; Ved, end-diastolic left ventricular volume; Ves, end-systolic left ventricular volume. (*Data from* Luecke T, Pelosi P. Clinical review: Positive end-expiratory pressure and cardiac output. Crit Care. 2005;9(6):607–21.)

In Predominantly Preload-Dependent State (= More Sensitive to Left Ventricular Preload, eg, Normal-Healthy Heart, Severe Right Ventricular Failure, or Under High Positive End-Expiratory Pressure)

PAP decreases VR and RV preload by elevating intrathoracic pressure, similarly to those in afterload-dependent state.[44] Increased intrathoracic pressure is transmitted to the pulmonary arteries; subsequently, the intraalveolar vessels become compressed. The compressed capillaries are lengthened and narrowed, leading to increased PVR (ie, increased RV afterload). Thus, both the decreased RV preload and the increased RV afterload have the net impact of diminishing the RV stroke volume.[36] Perceptibly, if there is a decrease in the RV stroke volume, there will also be a decrease in LV preload. PAP also can reduce LV afterload, in the same manner as in the afterload-dependent state. Therefore, the net balance of the

effects of PAP in the predominantly preload-dependent hemodynamic state leads to decreased LV stroke volume, resulting in decreased cardiac output (**Fig. 2**B). This phenomenon is also observed in patients with severe RV failure, Fontan circulation, or tamponade. Thus, PAP should be avoided if possible or should be used cautiously, in such patients. Importantly, because of high PEEP, the hemodynamic reaction provided by PAP in the afterload-dependent state may change to those in the preload-dependent state. Therefore, it is important to titrate the PEEP appropriately to avoid too much reduction in LV preload. In other words, "more than enough is too much."

INDICATION OF POSITIVE AIRWAY PRESSURE THERAPY FOR PATIENTS WITH ACUTE DECOMPENSATED HEART FAILURE

The therapeutic goals in the treatment of patients with cardiogenic pulmonary edema are to improve systemic oxygen saturation and stabilize hemodynamics as quickly as possible. PAP devices have great benefits for the patients because they can provide rapid improvement in gas exchange and normalize hemodynamics,[45–47] which can decrease the need for endotracheal intubation with the associated potential complications and clinical mortalities.[31,48] Guidelines for ADHF recommend using PAP devices before considering invasive ventilation if the patient with heart failure presents with symptoms of pulmonary edema or hypoxia despite supplying adequate oxygen.[3,26–28,49] The selection criteria and determinants of success for NIPPV are shown in **Box 1**.[50,51]

CONTRAINDICATION AND COMPLICATIONS OF POSITIVE AIRWAY PRESSURE DEVICES

CPAP should not be used in patients with inadequate spontaneous breathing. Patients with poor respiratory drive require invasive ventilation or noninvasive ventilation with CPAP plus additional pressure support and a backup rate. Therefore, bilevel PAP will be a good indication for those patients. The relative contraindications for NIPPV are shown in **Box 2**.[52]

Many complications have been reported in patients who undergo mechanical ventilation, including laryngotracheal injury, vocal cord paralysis, subglottic stenosis, and acquired aspiration pnemonitis.[48] In contrast, PAP devices are relatively safe and less subject to major complications.[53] Minor complications of PAP therapy are shown in **Box 2**.[48,54] If the mask is kept too tight for a long time, patients may suffer from skin lesions, especially on the nasal bridge.[55,56] Given that even any small discomfort or minor complications can cause reduced compliance, careful instructions must be given to patients.

TYPES AND CHARACTERISTICS OF POSITIVE AIRWAY PRESSURE DEVICES

There are several types of PAP devices. CPAP can maintain the constant PAP,[57] and the NIPPV devices, including bilevel PAP and ASV, are supplied by using a combination of pressure support ventilation and PEEP. PAP devices have a favorable potential to improve oxygenation and normalize abnormal respiratory patterns, provide pulmonary recruitment, and increase functional residual lung capacity. It can also provide decreased RV preload and afterload, decreased LV afterload, eventually to stabilize hemodynamics.[58] A summary of functions, advantages, and disadvantages in each NIPPV device is shown in **Table 2**.

Box 1
Selection criteria and determinants of success for noninvasive positive pressure ventilation in the acute setting

Selection criteria for NIPPV in the acute setting

Appropriate diagnosis with potential reversibility

Establish need for ventilatory assistance

    Moderate to severe respiratory distress

    Tachypnea

    Accessory muscle use or abdominal paradox

    Blood gas derangement: pH less than 7.35, $Paco_2$ greater than 45 mm Hg, or Pao_2/Fio_2 less than 200

Exclude patients with contraindications to NIPPV

    Respiratory arrest

    Medically unstable

    Unable to protect airway

    Excessive secretions

    Uncooperative or agitated

    Unable to fit mask

    Recent upper airway or gastrointestinal surgery

Determinants of success for NIPPV in the acute setting

Synchronous breathing

Dentition intact

Lower APACHE score

Less air leaking

Less secretions

    Good initial response to NIPPV

    Correction of pH

    Reduction of pH

    Reduction in respiratory rate

    Reduction in $Paco_2$

No pneumonia

    pH greater than 7.1

    $Paco_2$ less than 92 mm Hg

    Better neurologic score

    Better compliance

From Liesching T, Kwok H, Hill NS. Acute applications of noninvasive positive pressure ventilation. Chest. 2003;124(2):707–8; with permission.

Box 2
Relative contraindication and complications of noninvasive positive pressure ventilation

Relative contraindication of NIPPV

Difficult to cooperate to apply NIPPV

Unstable cardiorespiratory status

Patients with extremely anxiety

Poor consciousness

Unstable cardiorespiratory status

High risk of aspiration

Excessive secretions

Severe nausea with vomiting

Respiratory arrest

Anatomic abnormalities, including trauma or burns

After surgery of face, esophagus, and stomach

Air leak syndrome including pneumothorax

Skin lesion around mask area

Severe air trapping diseases, including asthma or chronic obstructive pulmonary disease

Severe right-side heart failure

Complications of NIPPV

Oral dryness

Eye irritation

Nasal congestion

Drooling

Sinus pain

Gastric distention

Skin lesion: transient erythema, skin ulceration, skin necrosis, especially at the nasal bridge

Pulmonary barotrauma (rare)

Continuous Positive Airway Pressure

CPAP is commonly used in patients with heart failure. CPAP can provide constant PAP support over the respiratory cycle (**Fig. 3**A). CPAP does not increase pressure during inspiration, so CPAP seems not to be classified as an NIPPV device. However, the international consensus conference in intensive care medicine defined an NIPPV device as any type of PAP device without endotracheal intubation.[52] Hence, CPAP is classified as a device of NIPPV in this review.

In patients with cardiogenic pulmonary edema, CPAP can provide positive thoracic pressure resulting in reduced VR and taking an advantage in LV transmural pressure and afterload, which will improve hemodynamics.[10,21,59] So far, clinical studies have demonstrated that CPAP was able to improve hypoxia, hypercapnia, and endotracheal intubation rates in patients with cardiogenic pulmonary edema, as compared with standard respiratory support (ie, oxygen by mask).[18,31,59–62] The mortality of those patients was improved by the CPAP in several clinical trials,[61,63,64] but not in others.[18,31,62] There was controversy regarding the impact of CPAP on mortality in those patients, but metaanalyses examined the effect on mortality.[65–67] In a metaanalysis of 13 trials, CPAP had a lower mortality than those with standard care alone.[66] A metaanalysis with 32 clinical studies revealed that NIPPV, including CPAP and bilevel PAP, significantly reduced hospital mortality in patients with cardiogenic pulmonary edema, compared with standard medical care.[67] The level of CPAP used in the clinical trials had diversity, but most of them used 10 cm H_2O for the CPAP level.[18,31,60,61,63,64] The titration of CPAP level is necessary for patient demand and comfort, whereas CPAP levels of 8.0 to 12.0 cm H_2O are the most appropriate levels used in the clinical setting.

Bilevel Positive Airway Pressure

Bilevel PAP can deliver both inspiratory positive airway pressure (IPAP) and expiratory positive airway pressure (EPAP), and it has physiologic advantages to CPAP through application of EPAP (**Fig. 3**B).[68] IPAP can be advantageous in providing alveolar recruitment, avoiding atelectatic alveoli, providing clearance of CO_2, and increasing lung functional residual capacity.[16] In addition, the EPAP can contribute to favorable effects, similar to hemodynamics changes provided by CPAP. Taken together, the bilevel PAP can improve both gas exchange and hemodynamics.[69–71] There are some differences in the actual airway support pressure between CPAP and bilevel PAP. In CPAP, the IPAP is lower than the applied CPAP level during inspiration, and the EPAP is higher (**Fig. 3**A). The CPAP during expiration can sometimes lead to difficulties in breathing, which can be associated with tolerance for the CPAP. In contrast to CPAP, in the bilevel PAP, the IPAP is greater than EPAP, reflecting the applied pressure support levels, and positive pressure support over respiratory cycle is maintained through the difference between IPAP and EPAP. Those properties in bilevel PAP can contribute to greater cardiac unloading effects and reduction of accumulated CO_2.[68] Therefore, the bilevel PAP may be a more acceptable therapeutic option for the treatment of cardiogenic pulmonary edema, compared with CPAP.

Table 2
Summary of functions, advantages, and disadvantages in each noninvasive positive pressure ventilation device

	CPAP	Bilevel PAP	ASV
Device function and properties			
PEEP	+	+	+
CO_2 clearance	+	++	−/+
Cardiac unloading	+	++	+
Pressure support during inspiration	−	+	+
Minimal ventilation	−	+	+
Backup ventilation		+	+
Servo control of ventilation	−	−	+
Advantages	Simple to use the device, less expensive, avoids incidence of endotracheal Intubation	Powerful improvement in oxygenation and CO_2 clearance, greater reduction in the workload of breathing, promoting alveolar ventilation, provides mandatory respiratory support, avoids incidence of endotracheal intubation	Comfortable, good tolerability, dynamically adjusts adequate support pressure, synchronizes and stabilizes patient's breathing, reduces sympathetic nerve activity, avoids Incidence of endotracheal intubation
Disadvantages	Minimal support, no ventilation support, IPAP is lower and EPAP is higher than the applied CPAP level during inspiration	Sometimes uncomfortable due to square shape pressure waveform	More expansive, less powerful compared with bilevel PAP (trade-off for comfort)

In the 3CPO trial, NIPPV, including CPAP (5–15 cm H_2O) or bilevel PAP (IPAP: 8–20, EPAP: 4–10 cm H_2O), could improve respiratory distress in comparison to standard O_2 therapy, but had no significant difference in the short-term mortality in patients with cardiogenic pulmonary edema.[18] A metaanalysis demonstrated that bilevel PAP was associated with avoiding intubation (relative risk [RR] = 0.54, 95% confidence interval [CI] 0.33–0.86) and a trend toward improved mortality, but not statistical significant (RR = 0.82, 95% CI 0.58–1.15), compared with standard care alone.[66] In another metaanalysis, NIPPV could reduce the need for intubation and reduce mortality in those patients, but there were no significant differences in clinical outcomes between CPAP and bilevel PAP.[72]

Adaptive Servoventilation

ASV is a novel NIPPV therapy that can provide automatically varying IPAP and EPAP, following the patient's spontaneous breathing pattern on demand, which leads to stabilized breathing (**Fig. 3**C).[73,74] Originally, ASV was developed for the treatment of Cheyne-Stokes respiration with central sleep apnea syndrome in patients with heart failure.[74] Owing to those novel functions, in addition to benefits of PAP, ASV can provide "comfortable" pressure support, which can contribute to decreased sympathetic nerve activity in the patient with heart failure.[22,23] Because patients with heart failure present a state of highly activated sympathetic nerve activity, which has implications for heart failure progression and its mortality,[75–78] the reduction in activated sympathetic nerve activity can be advantageous in the exertion of sympathoinhibitory effects and the reduction in RV/LV afterload.[22,23,73]

In Japan, ASV has been used for patients with ADHF in the emergency setting. Previous works have elucidated the acute and chronic

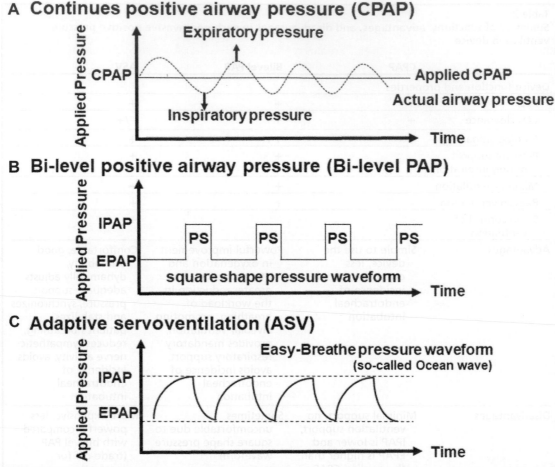

Fig. 3. Differences in applied pressure between CPAP, bilevel PAP, and ASV. (*A*) CPAP provides a constant level of PAP to avoid collapsed alveoli during spontaneous breathing. The IPAP is lower than the applied CPAP level during inspiration, and the EPAP is higher. (*B*) Bilevel PAP provides the 2 fixed levels of IPAP and EPAP. Bilevel PAP enables pressure support during inspiration, whereas CPAP cannot provide it. (*C*) ASV can automatically adjust the adequate pressure support for breath-by-breath demands, eventually synchronizing and stabilizing breathing patterns. PS, pressure support. (*Data from* Refs.[68,73,74])

effects of ASV on hemodynamics and mortality.[22,23,42,73,79–84] As ASV exerts an acute impact on hemodynamics, there is reduction of LV afterload resulting in an increase of stroke volume and cardiac output.[73,79,80] Higher LVEDP, severity of mitral regurgitation, and LV spherical shape index are independent predictors for acute beneficial effects of ASV on hemodynamics.[80] ASV can improve the short-term prognosis and fatal cardiovascular events in patients with heart failure, regardless of sleep-disordered breathing severity.[81,82] In the SAVIOR-C trial, ASV therapy did not have superiority to guideline-directed medical therapy in the improvement of cardiac function, but revealed a clinical status-improving effect.[83] There were negative randomized controlled trials related to the impact of ASV on mortality.[85–88] Given that higher IPAP or EPAP

might be applied in order to completely treat the sleep apnea syndrome, as a result, the hemodynamic improvement effect by ASV may be eventually spoiled. Therefore, "pure" potential benefits of ASV on hemodynamics and mortality remain to be confirmed.

SUMMARY

The pathophysiology of patients with cardiogenic pulmonary edema is associated with pulmonary vascular congestion and excessive alveolar fluid, which can lead to arterial hypoxemia, reduced lung compliance, and increased PVR. Both the liquid-filled alveoli and the high PVR will be a trigger to the vicious cycle of the cardiogenic pulmonary edema. For cardiovascular emergencies, the NIPPV devices can provide favorable effects not only to the pulmonary system but also to the systemic hemodynamics. PAP therapy can recruit collapsed alveoli and increase lung functional residual capacity, thereby decreasing breathing workload, but it also can decrease RV preload/afterload and LV afterload. The hemodynamic net effect of PEEP on cardiac output depends on both RV and LV functions, preload, and afterload; therefore, elucidating the hemodynamics and cardiac functions is paramount.

ACKNOWLEDGMENTS

The author sincerely thanks Drs Yogamaya Mantha, Danilo Cardim, and Rakushumimarika Harada as English editors of the final manuscript submitted for publication.

DISCLOSURE

The author has nothing to disclose.

REFERENCES

1. Benjamin EJ, Blaha MJ, Chiuve SE, et al. Heart disease and stroke statistics–2017 update: a report from the American Heart Association. Circulation 2017;135(10):e146–603.
2. Heidenreich PA, Albert NM, Allen LA, et al. Forecasting the impact of heart failure in the United States: a policy statement from the American Heart Association. Circ Heart Fail 2013;6(3):606–19.
3. Yancy CW, Jessup M, Bozkurt B, et al. 2013 ACCF/AHA guideline for the management of heart failure: executive summary. A report of the American College of Cardiology Foundation/American Heart Association Task Force on Practice Guidelines. Circulation 2013;62(16):1495–539.
4. Crespo-Leiro MG, Metra M, Lund LH, et al. Advanced heart failure: a position statement of the Heart Failure Association of the European Society of Cardiology. Eur J Heart Fail 2018;20(11):1505–35.
5. Friedrich EB, Böhm M. Management of end stage heart failure. Heart 2007;93(5):626–31.
6. Cleland JG, Gemmell I, Khand A, et al. Is the prognosis of heart failure improving? Eur J Heart Fail 1999;1(3):229–41.
7. Allen LA, Stevenson LW, Grady KL, et al. Decision making in advanced heart failure: a scientific statement from the American Heart Association. Circulation 2012;125(15):1928–52.
8. Poulton EP. Left-sided heart failure with pulmonary oedema: its treatment with the "pulmonary plus pressure machine". Lancet 1936;228(5904):981–3.
9. Bello G, De Santis P, Antonelli M. Non-invasive ventilation in cardiogenic pulmonary edema. Ann Transl Med 2018;6(18):355.
10. Bradley TD, Holloway RM, McLaughlin PR, et al. Cardiac output response to continuous positive airway pressure in congestive heart failure. Am Rev Respir Dis 1992;145(2 Pt 1):377–82.
11. Pang D, Keenan SP, Cook DJ, et al. The effect of positive pressure airway support on mortality and the need for intubation in cardiogenic pulmonary edema: a systematic review. Chest 1998;114(4):1185–92.
12. Parsons CL, Sole ML, Byers JF. Noninvasive positive-pressure ventilation: averting intubation of the heart failure patient. Dimens Crit Care Nurs 2000;19(6):18–24.
13. Wigder HN, Hoffmann P, Mazzolini D, et al. Pressure support noninvasive positive pressure ventilation treatment of acute cardiogenic pulmonary edema. Am J Emerg Med 2001;19(3):179–81.
14. L'Her E. Noninvasive mechanical ventilation in acute cardiogenic pulmonary edema. Curr Opin Crit Care 2003;9(1):67–71.
15. Agarwal R, Aggarwal AN, Gupta D, et al. Non-invasive ventilation in acute cardiogenic pulmonary oedema. Postgrad Med J 2005;81(960):637–43.
16. Park M, Lorenzi-Filho G. Noninvasive mechanical ventilation in the treatment of acute cardiogenic pulmonary edema. Clinics (Sao Paulo) 2006;61(3):247–52.
17. Ursella S, Mazzone M, Portale G, et al. The use of non-invasive ventilation in the treatment of acute cardiogenic pulmonary edema. Eur Rev Med Pharmacol Sci 2007;11(3):193–205.
18. Gray A, Goodacre S, Newby DE, et al. Noninvasive ventilation in acute cardiogenic pulmonary edema. N Engl J Med 2008;359(2):142–51.
19. Berbenetz N, Wang Y, Brown J, et al. Non-invasive positive pressure ventilation (CPAP or bilevel NPPV) for cardiogenic pulmonary oedema. Cochrane Database Syst Rev 2019;(4):CD005351.
20. Theerakittikul T, Ricaurte B, Aboussouan LS. Noninvasive positive pressure ventilation for stable outpatients: CPAP and beyond. Cleve Clin J Med 2010;77(10):705–14.
21. Kato T, Suda S, Kasai T. Positive airway pressure therapy for heart failure. World J Cardiol 2014;6(11):1175–91.
22. Harada D, Joho S, Oda Y, et al. Short term effect of adaptive servo-ventilation on muscle sympathetic nerve activity in patients with heart failure. Auton Neurosci 2011;161(1–2):95–102.
23. Joho S, Oda Y, Ushijima R, et al. Effect of adaptive servoventilation on muscle sympathetic nerve activity in patients with chronic heart failure and central sleep apnea. J Card Fail 2012;18(10):769–75.
24. Gheorghiade M, Zannad F, Sopko G, et al. Acute heart failure syndromes: current state and framework for future research. Circulation 2005;112(25):3958–68.

25. Weintraub Neal L, Collins Sean P, Pang Peter S, et al. Acute heart failure syndromes: emergency department presentation, treatment, and disposition: current approaches and future aims. Circulation 2010;122(19):1975–96.

26. Ponikowski P, Voors AA, Anker SD, et al. 2016 ESC Guidelines for the diagnosis and treatment of acute and chronic heart failure: the Task Force for the diagnosis and treatment of acute and chronic heart failure of the European Society of Cardiology (ESC). Developed with the special contribution of the Heart Failure Association (HFA) of the ESC. Eur J Heart Fail 2016;18(8):891–975.

27. Yancy CW, Jessup M, Bozkurt B, et al. 2017 ACC/AHA/HFSA focused update of the 2013 ACCF/AHA guideline for the management of heart failure: a report of the American College of Cardiology/American Heart Association Task Force on Clinical Practice Guidelines and the Heart Failure Society of America. Circulation 2017;136(6):e137–61.

28. Tsutsui H, Isobe M, Ito H, et al. JCS 2017/JHFS 2017 guideline on diagnosis and treatment of acute and chronic heart failure- digest version. Circ J 2019; 83(10):2084–184.

29. Sharp JT, Griffith GT, Bunnell IL, et al. Ventilatory mechanics in pulmonary edema in man. J Clin Invest 1958;37(1):111–7.

30. Luisada AA, Cardi L. Acute pulmonary edema; pathology, physiology and clinical management. Circulation 1956;13(1):113–35.

31. Bersten AD, Holt AW, Vedig AE, et al. Treatment of severe cardiogenic pulmonary edema with continuous positive airway pressure delivered by face mask. N Engl J Med 1991;325(26):1825–30.

32. Staub NC. Pulmonary edema. Physiol Rev 1974; 54(3):678–811.

33. Ware LB, Matthay MA. Clinical practice. Acute pulmonary edema. N Engl J Med 2005;353(26): 2788–96.

34. Milne EN, Pistolesi M, Miniati M, et al. The radiologic distinction of cardiogenic and noncardiogenic edema. AJR Am J Roentgenol 1985;144(5): 879–94.

35. Perlman CE, Lederer DJ, Bhattacharya J. Micromechanics of alveolar edema. Am J Respir Cell Mol Biol 2011;44(1):34–9.

36. Cassidy SS, Mitchell JH. Effects of positive pressure breathing on right and left ventricular preload and afterload. Fed Proc 1981;40(8):2178–81.

37. Alviar CL, Miller PE, McAreavey D, et al. Positive pressure ventilation in the cardiac intensive care unit. J Am Coll Cardiol 2018;72(13):1532–53.

38. Duke GJ. Cardiovascular effects of mechanical ventilation. Crit Care Resusc 1999;1(4):388–99.

39. Reddi B, Shanmugam N, Fletcher N. Heart failure—pathophysiology and inpatient management. BJA Educ 2017;17(5):151–60.

40. Luce JM. The cardiovascular effects of mechanical ventilation and positive end-expiratory pressure. JAMA 1984;252(6):807–11.

41. Frenneaux M, Williams L. Ventricular-arterial and ventricular-ventricular interactions and their relevance to diastolic filling. Prog Cardiovasc Dis 2007;49(4):252–62.

42. Hieda M, Seguchi O, Mutara Y, et al. Acute response test to adaptive servo-ventilation, a possible modality to assessing the reversibility of pulmonary vascular resistance. J Artif Organs 2015;18(3):280–3.

43. Luecke T, Pelosi P. Clinical review: positive end-expiratory pressure and cardiac output. Crit Care 2005;9(6):607–21.

44. Cassidy SS, Eschenbacher WL, Robertson CH Jr, et al. Cardiovascular effects of positive-pressure ventilation in normal subjects. J Appl Physiol Respir Environ Exerc Physiol 1979;47(2):453–61.

45. Rasanen J, Heikkila J, Downs J, et al. Continuous positive airway pressure by face mask in acute cardiogenic pulmonary edema. Am J Cardiol 1985; 55(4):296–300.

46. Masip J, Betbese AJ, Paez J, et al. Non-invasive pressure support ventilation versus conventional oxygen therapy in acute cardiogenic pulmonary oedema: a randomised trial. Lancet 2000; 356(9248):2126–32.

47. Nava S, Carbone G, DiBattista N, et al. Noninvasive ventilation in cardiogenic pulmonary edema: a multicenter randomized trial. Am J Respir Crit Care Med 2003;168(12):1432–7.

48. Brochard L. Mechanical ventilation: invasive versus noninvasive. Eur Respir J Suppl 2003;47:31s–7s.

49. Collins SP, Storrow AB, Levy PD, et al. Early management of patients with acute heart failure: state of the art and future directions–a consensus document from the SAEM/HFSA Acute Heart Failure Working Group. Acad Emerg Med 2015;22(1): 94–112.

50. Liesching T, Kwok H, Hill NS. Acute applications of noninvasive positive pressure ventilation. Chest 2003;124(2):699–713.

51. Shirakabe A, Hata N, Yokoyama S, et al. Predicting the success of noninvasive positive pressure ventilation in emergency room for patients with acute heart failure. J Cardiol 2011;57(1):107–14.

52. International Consensus Conferences in Intensive Care Medicine: noninvasive positive pressure ventilation in acute respiratory failure. Am J Respir Crit Care Med 2001;163(1):283–91.

53. Winck JC, Azevedo LF, Costa-Pereira A, et al. Efficacy and safety of non-invasive ventilation in the treatment of acute cardiogenic pulmonary edema– a systematic review and meta-analysis. Crit Care 2006;10(2):R69.

54. Carron M, Freo U, BaHammam AS, et al. Complications of non-invasive ventilation techniques: a

comprehensive qualitative review of randomized trials. Br J Anaesth 2013;110(6):896–914.

55. Visscher MO, White CC, Jones JM, et al. Face masks for noninvasive ventilation: fit, excess skin hydration, and pressure ulcers. Respir Care 2015; 60(11):1536–47.

56. Fauroux B, Lavis JF, Nicot F, et al. Facial side effects during noninvasive positive pressure ventilation in children. Intensive Care Med 2005;31(7):965–9.

57. Masip J. Noninvasive ventilation in acute heart failure. Curr Heart Fail Rep 2019;16(4):89–97.

58. Peter JV, Moran JL, Phillips-Hughes J, et al. Effect of non-invasive positive pressure ventilation (NIPPV) on mortality in patients with acute cardiogenic pulmonary oedema: a meta-analysis. Lancet 2006; 367(9517):1155–63.

59. Dib JE, Matin SA, Luckert A. Prehospital use of continuous positive airway pressure for acute severe congestive heart failure. J Emerg Med 2012;42(5): 553–8.

60. Lin M, Yang YF, Chiang HT, et al. Reappraisal of continuous positive airway pressure therapy in acute cardiogenic pulmonary edema. Short-term results and long-term follow-up. Chest 1995;107(5): 1379–86.

61. L'Her E, Duquesne F, Girou E, et al. Noninvasive continuous positive airway pressure in elderly cardiogenic pulmonary edema patients. Intensive Care Med 2004;30(5):882–8.

62. Kulkarni VT, Kim N, Dai Y, et al. Hospital variation in noninvasive positive pressure ventilation for acute decompensated heart failure. Circ Heart Fail 2014; 7(3):427–33.

63. Crane SD, Elliott MW, Gilligan P, et al. Randomised controlled comparison of continuous positive airways pressure, bilevel non-invasive ventilation, and standard treatment in emergency department patients with acute cardiogenic pulmonary oedema. Emerg Med J 2004;21(2):155–61.

64. Park M, Sangean MC, Volpe Mde S, et al. Randomized, prospective trial of oxygen, continuous positive airway pressure, and bilevel positive airway pressure by face mask in acute cardiogenic pulmonary edema. Crit Care Med 2004;32(12):2407–15.

65. Potts JM. Noninvasive positive pressure ventilation: effect on mortality in acute cardiogenic pulmonary edema: a pragmatic meta-analysis. Pol Arch Med Wewn 2009;119(6):349–53.

66. Weng CL, Zhao YT, Liu QH, et al. Meta-analysis: noninvasive ventilation in acute cardiogenic pulmonary edema. Ann Intern Med 2010;152(9):590–600.

67. Vital FM, Ladeira MT, Atallah AN. Non-invasive positive pressure ventilation (CPAP or bilevel NPPV) for cardiogenic pulmonary oedema. Cochrane Database Syst Rev 2013;(5):CD005351.

68. Murray S. Bi-level positive airway pressure (BiPAP) and acute cardiogenic pulmonary oedema (ACPO)

in the emergency department. Aust Crit Care 2002; 15(2):51–63.

69. Kuhn BT, Bradley LA, Dempsey TM, et al. Management of mechanical ventilation in decompensated heart failure. J Cardiovasc Dev Dis 2016;3(4):33.

70. Pinsky MR. The effects of mechanical ventilation on the cardiovascular system. Crit Care Clin 1990;6(3): 663–78.

71. Shekerdemian L, Bohn D. Cardiovascular effects of mechanical ventilation. Arch Dis Child 1999;80(5): 475–80.

72. Masip J, Roque M, Sanchez B, et al. Noninvasive ventilation in acute cardiogenic pulmonary edema: systematic review and meta-analysis. JAMA 2005; 294(24):3124–30.

73. Asakawa N, Sakakibara M, Noguchi K, et al. Adaptive servo-ventilation has more favorable acute effects on hemodynamics than continuous positive airway pressure in patients with heart failure. Int Heart J 2015;56(5):527–32.

74. Teschler H, Dohring J, Wang YM, et al. Adaptive pressure support servo-ventilation: a novel treatment for Cheyne-Stokes respiration in heart failure. Am J Respir Crit Care Med 2001;164(4):614–9.

75. Floras JS. Sympathetic nervous system activation in human heart failure: clinical implications of an updated model. J Am Coll Cardiol 2009;54(5):375–85.

76. Cohn JN, Levine TB, Olivari MT, et al. Plasma norepinephrine as a guide to prognosis in patients with chronic congestive heart failure. N Engl J Med 1984;311(13):819–23.

77. Triposkiadis F, Karayannis G, Giamouzis G, et al. The sympathetic nervous system in heart failure physiology, pathophysiology, and clinical implications. J Am Coll Cardiol 2009;54(19):1747–62.

78. Kaye DM, Lefkovits J, Jennings GL, et al. Adverse consequences of high sympathetic nervous activity in the failing human heart. J Am Coll Cardiol 1995; 26(5):1257–63.

79. Haruki N, Takeuchi M, Kaku K, et al. Comparison of acute and chronic impact of adaptive servo-ventilation on left chamber geometry and function in patients with chronic heart failure. Eur J Heart Fail 2011;13(10):1140–6.

80. Yamada S, Sakakibara M, Yokota T, et al. Acute hemodynamic effects of adaptive servo-ventilation in patients with heart failure. Circ J 2013;77(5):1214–20.

81. Koyama T, Watanabe H, Igarashi G, et al. Short-term prognosis of adaptive servo-ventilation therapy in patients with heart failure. Circ J 2011;75(3):710–2.

82. Takama N, Kurabayashi M. Effect of adaptive servo-ventilation on 1-year prognosis in heart failure patients. Circ J 2012;76(3):661–7.

83. Momomura S, Seino Y, Kihara Y, et al. Adaptive servo-ventilation therapy for patients with chronic heart failure in a confirmatory, multicenter, randomized, controlled study. Circ J 2015;79(5):981–90.

84. Momomura S, Seino Y, Kihara Y, et al. Adaptive servo-ventilation therapy using an innovative ventilator for patients with chronic heart failure: a real-world, multicenter, retrospective, observational study (SAVIOR-R). Heart Vessels 2015;30(6): 805–17.

85. Arzt M, Floras JS, Logan AG, et al. Suppression of central sleep apnea by continuous positive airway pressure and transplant-free survival in heart failure: a post hoc analysis of the Canadian Continuous Positive Airway Pressure for Patients with Central Sleep Apnea and Heart Failure Trial (CANPAP). Circulation 2007;115(25):3173–80.

86. Bradley TD, Logan AG, Kimoff RJ, et al. Continuous positive airway pressure for central sleep apnea and heart failure. N Engl J Med 2005;353(19): 2025–33.

87. Cowie MR, Woehrle H, Wegscheider K, et al. Adaptive servo-ventilation for central sleep apnea in systolic heart failure. N Engl J Med 2015;373(12): 1095–105.

88. O'Connor CM, Whellan DJ, Fiuzat M, et al. Cardiovascular outcomes with minute ventilation-targeted adaptive servo-ventilation therapy in heart failure: the CAT-HF trial. J Am Coll Cardiol 2017;69(12): 1577–87.

How to Manage Temporary Mechanical Circulatory Support Devices in the Critical Care Setting
Translating Physiology to the Bedside

Prashant Rao, MD[a],*, Daniel Katz, MD[a], Michinari Hieda, MD, MSc, PhD[b],
Marwa Sabe, MD, MPH[a]

KEYWORDS

- Cardiogenic shock • Mechanical circulatory support devices • Acute myocardial infarction

KEY POINTS

- A deep understanding of the pathophysiology of cardiogenic shock can be reached through basic hemodynamic and myocardial energetic principles.
- It is important to understand the forms of temporary mechanical circulatory support, their advantages, disadvantages and practical considerations relating to implementation and management.
- The different platforms for temporary mechanical circulatory support should all be considered as part of a physician's toolkit, rather than a 'one-size-fits-all' approach.
- It is through the translation of underlying physiologic principles that we can attempt to maximize the clinical utility of circulatory support devices and improve outcomes in cardiogenic shock.

INTRODUCTION

Cardiogenic shock (CS) is a low cardiac output state causing life-threatening end-organ hypoperfusion and hypoxemia.[1–3] Although it is difficult to determine the true incidence of CS, both the proportion of intensive care unit admissions with CS and the number of US discharges complicated by CS have doubled over the past 15 years.[4,5] Acute myocardial infarction (AMI) remains the most common cause for CS. Of all patients with AMI, CS occurs in 8% to 9% of those with an ST-segment elevation myocardial infarction, and 2.5% of patients with a non-ST-segment myocardial infarction.[6,7] Despite advances in medical therapies and coronary revascularization, CS portends a poor prognosis with in-hospital mortality between 27% and 51%.[7–9] In this review, we discuss the cause and pathophysiology of CS as well as its attendant hemodynamic changes. We also explore the various mechanical circulatory support mechanical circulatory support (MCS) platforms available to treat CS and provide a framework for deciding the optimal MCS device for any given patient with CS.

Funding: M. Hieda was supported in part by the American Heart Association Strategically Focused Research Network (14SFRN20600009-03). Dr M. Hieda was also supported by American Heart Association postdoctoral fellowship grant (18POST33960092) and the Harry S. Moss Heart Trust. D. Katz was supported by a National Institutes of Health grant (5T32HL007374-40).

a Beth Israel Deaconess Medical Center, Harvard Medical School, Boston, MA, USA; b University of Texas Southwestern Medical Center, Institute for Exercise and Environmental Medicine, Texas Health Presbyterian Hospital Dallas, 7232 Greenville Avenue, Dallas, TX 75231, USA
* Corresponding author. 330 Brookline Avenue, Baker 4th Floor, Boston, MA 02215.
E-mail address: prao@bidmc.harvard.edu
Twitter: @DrPRao (P.R.)

Heart Failure Clin 16 (2020) 283–293
https://doi.org/10.1016/j.hfc.2020.03.001
1551-7136/20/© 2020 Elsevier Inc. All rights reserved.

THE PATHOPHYSIOLOGY OF CARDIOGENIC SHOCK
Cause

Classically, the most common cause of CS is AMI. However, there are multiple dysfunctional states that can result in a cardiac output that is inadequate to support end-organ function. These common causes of CS are summarized in **Box 1**.

Progression of Cardiogenic Shock

Cardiac dysfunction from any cause frequently begets further cardiac dysfunction. The initial drop in cardiac output from the primary insult leads to decreased coronary perfusion, creating or enhancing myocardial ischemia, and eventually may lead to systolic and diastolic cardiac dysfunction. At the same time, cardiac dysfunction results in pulmonary edema, which reduces global oxygen supply. Decreased perfusion also causes vascular dysfunction and inflammation, ultimately leading to an imbalance of preload and afterload. These mechanisms form a negative feedback loop of progressive dysfunction that spirals toward end-organ failure and eventually death if timely intervention is not pursued.

THE HEMODYNAMICS OF CARDIOGENIC SHOCK

A deeper understanding of the pathophysiologic cascade of CS can be reached through basic

---

Box 1
Cause of cardiogenic shock

Ischemic

- Acute coronary syndromes
- Hypoxemia or anemia in the setting of stable coronary disease

Structural

- Acute mitral regurgitation
- Critical aortic stenosis

Obstructive

- Cardiac tamponade
- Pulmonary embolism

Electrical

- Ventricular tachycardic storm

Cardiomyopathic

- Acute on chronic heart failure decompensation
- Myocarditis
- Septic cardiomyopathy

---

hemodynamic and myocardial energetic principles. The standard pressure-volume (PV) loop for a normal heart is shown in **Fig. 1**A. The end-systolic pressure volume relationship (ESPVR) represents the intrinsic systolic function of the heart. The slope of the ESPVR is an approximation of *contractility* and is known as the end-systolic elastance. The diastolic function of the heart is represented by the end-diastolic pressure volume relationship (EDPVR). The ESPVR and EDPVR are intrinsic to the myocardium, and as such, for any given preload or afterload, the specific PV loop assumed by the heart can change, but is bounded by the ESPVR and EDPVR. If a normal heart suffers an AMI, the expected shift is shown in **Fig. 1**B and is the result of an acute insult to intrinsic contractile function, manifesting specifically as a decrease in the slope of the ESPVR. The new PV loop demonstrates the increase in end-diastolic volume as well as the weakened contractile force that produces a smaller stroke volume. The energetics of this new state is an important factor in the ensuing downward spiral observed in CS.

Generally speaking, the heart consumes energy for 2 major purposes. The first is what is required to maintain its shape and electrical function, termed potential energy (PE), and the second is the energy used to actually pump blood, termed stroke work (SW). The area bounded by the ESPVR, EDPVR, and the PV loop measures the total required energy, which is directly proportional to the myocardial oxygen demand. Although the total required energy of the normal and total required energy of the acutely insulted heart are similar, in the latter, the proportion of total energy consumed by PE is greater with a concomitant reduction in SW (**Fig. 1**C, D). Because the SW is also proportional to myocardial oxygen supply, the acutely insulted heart can rapidly lead to imbalance in myocardial oxygen supply and demand, resulting in progressive ischemia and dysfunction.

Timely intervention in CS is critical to prevent the attendant downward spiral. The goal of intervention is to reverse the causative insult and correct the hemodynamic and energetic imbalances that propagate CS. For example, urgent reperfusion in AMI,[3] thrombolysis, or thrombectomy for massive pulmonary embolism, and possible immunosuppression for myocarditis are central to the management of these disease states when complicated by CS. At the same time, vasopressors and inotropes are frequently required for hemodynamic support. These agents are useful for rapid, short-term stabilization owing to their availability, rapid onset, and ease of initiation. However, inotropes increase myocardial oxygen

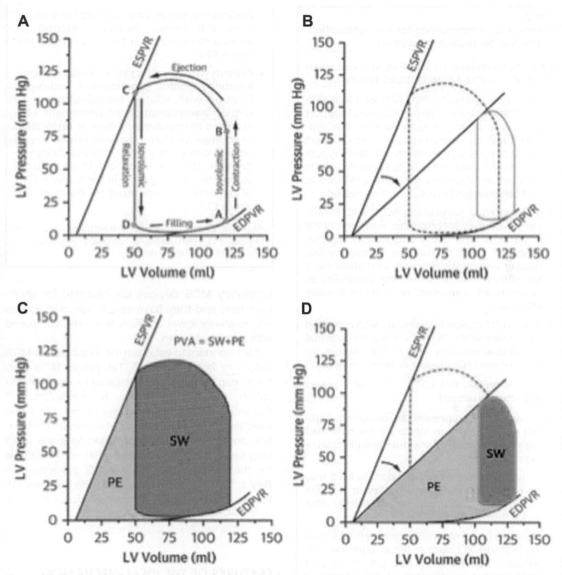

Fig. 1. (*A*) The standard PV loop for a normal heart. (*B*) In an acute insult, the systolic function decreases represented by a decrease in the slope of the ESPVR. (*C*) Components of the PV area, which is made up of the SW and the PE in a normal heart. (*D*) PE and SW during an acute cardiac insult. PVA, pressure volume area. (*Adapted from Uriel N, Sayer G, Annamalai S, et al. Mechanical unloading in heart failure. J Am Coll Cardiol. 2018;2072:569–580; with permission.*)

demand, whereas vasopressors may impair end-organ microcirculation. MCS devices are therefore useful in CS because they not only provide systemic circulatory support and end-organ perfusion but also can reduce myocardial oxygen demand and increase myocardial oxygen supply. Such myocardial energetics afforded by MCS devices may directly reverse the negative feedback look of CS and prevent the downward spiral toward death.[10]

KEY PRINCIPLES TO CONSIDER WHEN INITIATING TEMPORARY MECHANICAL CIRCULATORY SUPPORT

Escalation of doses of inotropes and vasopressors is associated with increased mortality.[11] MCS can help stabilize patients with CS and reduce the need for inotropes and vasopressors. The major difference between the temporary MCS and durable devices depends on the expected period requiring circulatory support. In general, the

---

Box 2
Current recommendations for implementation of mechanical circulatory support

2016 ESC Guidelines for the diagnosis and treatment of acute and chronic heart failure

- To manage patients with AHF or CS (INTERMACS level 1), short-term mechanical support systems, including percutaneous cardiac support devices, extracorporeal life support (ECLS) and extracorporeal membrane oxygenation (ECMO) may be used to support patients with left or biventricular failure until cardiac and other organ function have recovered.

- MCS systems, particularly ECLS and ECMO, can be used as a "bridge to decision" (BTD) in patients with acute and rapidly deteriorating HF or CS to stabilize hemodynamics, recover end-organ function, and allow for a full clinical evaluation for the possibility of either heart transplant or a more durable MCS device.

- A difficult decision to withdraw MCS may need to be made when the patient has no potential for cardiac recovery and is not eligible for longer-term MCS support or heart transplant.

2015 SCAI/ACC/HFSA/STS Clinical Expert Consensus Statement

- Patients in CS represent an extremely high-risk group in whom mortality has remained high despite revascularization and pharmacologic therapies.

- Early placement of an appropriate MCS may be considered in those who fail to stabilize or show signs of improvement quickly after initial interventions.

- MCS may be considered for patients undergoing high-risk PCI, such as those requiring multivessel, left main, or last patent conduit interventions, particularly if the patient is inoperable or has severely decreased ejection fraction or elevated cardiac filling pressures.

- MCS may be considered if patients are candidates for surgically implanted VADs or if rapid recovery is expected (eg, fulminant myocarditis or stress-induced cardiomyopathy).

HFSA comprehensive HF practice guidelines

- Patients awaiting heart transplantation who have become refractory to all means of medical circulatory support should be considered for an MCS device as a BTT (Level of Evidence B).

- Permanent mechanical assistance using an implantable assist device may be considered in highly selected patients with severe HF refractory to conventional therapy who are not candidates for heart transplantation,

particularly those who cannot be weaned from intravenous inotropic support at an experienced HF center (Strength of Evidence B)

- Patients with refractory HF and hemodynamic instability and/or compromised end-organ function with relative contraindications to cardiac transplantation or permanent MCS expected to improve with time or restoration of an improved hemodynamic profile should be considered for urgent MCS as a bridge to decision; these patients should be referred to a center with expertise in the management of patients with advanced HF (Level of Evidence C).

Abbreviations: BTT, bridge-to-transplant; HF, heart failure; PCI, percutaneous coronary intervention; VAD, ventricular assist device.

---

temporary MCS devices are intended for short-term use, and they have simple vascular access and relatively lower auxiliary flow rate, compared with durable devices.

It is important to establish the exact goal of MCS before its implementation. Temporary MCS platforms can be used as a bridge to recovery, destination therapy or bridge to transplant.[12–16] Recently, temporary MCS devices are also being used as a bridge to decision while further information about the patient is obtained to guide more long-term therapies. Current recommendations for the initiation of MCS for CS are shown in **Box 2**.[15–17] The authors also provide a framework to help with this decision-making process in **Fig. 2.**

FEATURES OF THE IDEAL MECHANICAL CIRCULATORY SUPPORT SYSTEM

The ideal MCS platform is able to perform 3 important hemodynamic functions. First, it should provide adequate circulatory support and systemic perfusion. Second, it should decrease left ventricular (LV) preload and afterload. Finally, it should increase coronary perfusion pressure through an increase in diastolic blood pressure (DBP) and/or decrease in LV end-diastolic pressure (LVEDP).[18,19] With regards to implementation, mechanical circulatory support should be easy and rapid to insert without high levels of expertise. Also, ideally they should be associated with low rates of known complications, including bleeding, stroke, infection, and limb ischemia, although these are well-known and often unavoidable complications of MCS (**Box 3**).[20–28]

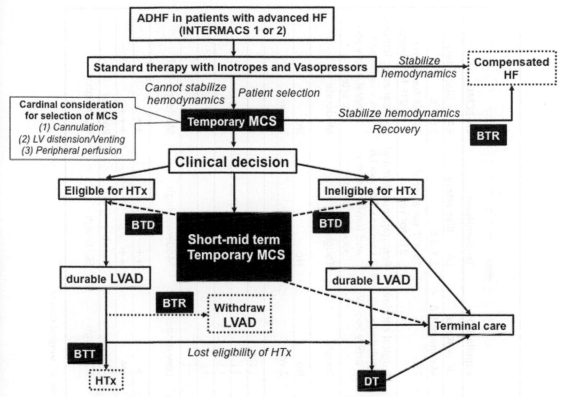

Fig. 2. Decision making framework for use of temporary MCS, durable devices, and heart transplant for patients with CS. LVAD, left ventricular assist device. ADHF, acute decompensated heart failure; BTD, bridge to destination; BTR, bridge to recovery; DT, destination therapy; HTx, heart transplant; LVAD, left ventricular assist device.

HOW TO SELECT THE APPROPRIATE TEMPORARY MECHANICAL CIRCULATORY SUPPORT SYSTEM

There are several forms of MCS devices that can be used to support patients with CS. The choice of MCS platform should take into consideration both patient and platform factors. Patient-related factors include their comorbidities, expected prognosis assuming cardiac recovery, and unique hemodynamic profile. Given that the choice of MCS is tailored according to the individual hemodynamic profile, right heart catheterization with a pulmonary artery catheter is critical for the management of these patients. The underlying cardiac substrate is also important to consider, whether the inciting injury was an index event in a previously normal heart or in the setting of chronic heart failure and dilated cardiomyopathy. Other important patient-related factors include the reversibility of the disease process and involvement of the right ventricle.

Each MCS device has distinct hemodynamic characteristics, different catheter sizes, and/or cannulas used, as well as blood drainage and return sites (**Table 1**). In addition, some platforms require percutaneous versus surgical implementation, and there are devices that provide gas exchange for patients with cardiac and respiratory failure. As mentioned in the previous section, the optimal MCS device should provide systemic

Box 3
Characteristics of the ideal mechanical circulatory support device
• Widely accessible
• Rapidly inserted via a minimally invasive approach
• Minimal bleeding and vascular /ischemic complications
• Provide immediate circulatory support
• Direct LV volume and pressure unloading
• Increase coronary perfusion pressure
• Provide gas exchange if needed
• Benign weaning and removal

Table 1
Technical properties of percutaneous circulatory assist devices

Feature	IABP	Impella 2.5	Impella CP	Impella 5.0	TandemHeart	VA-ECMO
Mechanism	Balloon pumping	LV → Aorta	LV → Aorta	LV → Aorta	LA → Iliac artery	RA → Iliac artery
Flow (L/min)	0.2–0.6	Maximum 2.5	Maximum 3.5	Maximum 5.0	2.5–5.0	3.0–7.0
Cannula size	8F	12F	14F	23F	15–17F for arterial 21F for venous	14–16F for arterial 18–21F for venous
Insertion	Percutaneous: femoral artery >>> descending aorta	Percutaneous: femoral artery >>> LV	Percutaneous: femoral artery >>> LV	Surgical cut down: subclavian artery >>> LV	Percutaneous: femoral vein >>> RA >>> LA and femoral artery >>> iliac artery	Percutaneous: femoral vein >>> RA and femoral artery >>> iliac artery
Setup and implementation	Very easy	Easy	Easy	Tough	Tough	Moderate
Cardiac synchrony	Yes	No	No	No	No	No
Maximum implant time	5–7 d	5–10 d	5–10 d	2 wk	2 wk	3–4 wk
Preload	No change	↓	↓	↓↓	↓↓	↓↓
LVEDP	↓	↓↓	↓↓	↓↓	↓↓	↑↑
LV afterload	↓	↓↓	↓↓	↓↓	↓↓	↑↑↑
Coronary perfusion	↑↑	↑	↑	↑	↑	→ or ↑
Peripheral perfusion	Slightly ↑	↑	↑	↑↑	↑↑	↑↑
Anticoagulation drug	Relatively low	Low-moderate	Low-moderate	Low-moderate	Moderate-high	Moderate-high
Hemolysis	−	+++	++	+	++	++
Limb ischemia	+	++	++	++	++	+++
Oxygenation	−	−	−	−	Possible	Possible
Exit strategy	Hand, manually, easy	SC, moderate	SC, moderate	SC, tough	SC, tough	SC, tough

Abbreviations: IVC, inferior vena cava; PA, pulmonary artery; RA, right atrium; RV, right ventricle; SC, surgical closure.

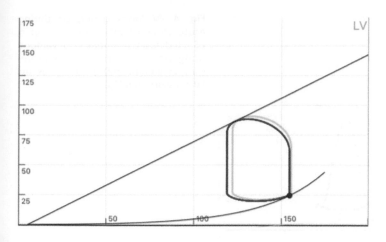

Fig. 3. PV loops generated during acute CS and IABP. Green loop = CS. Red loop = IABP. Developed using Harvi - online.[34] x-axis represents LV volume (ml); y-axis represents LV pressure (mmHg).

circulatory support, LV volume and pressure unloading, and coronary perfusion.

In the following section, we discuss the most common platforms for temporary MCS, their advantages and disadvantages, and practical considerations relating to implementation and management. These devices should all be considered as part of a physician's toolkit, rather than a "one-size-fits-all" approach.

INTRAAORTIC BALLOON PUMP

First used clinically in 1967,[29] the intraaortic balloon pump (IABP) is the most widely implemented MCS device, with around 50,000 devices implanted per year in the United States.[30] Its familiarity of use in clinical practice and relative ease of insertion explain the high implantation rate despite an increasing utilization of newer forms of MCS.

Hemodynamic Effects

In essence, the IABP provides counterpulsation: the balloon, which lies in the descending aorta, inflates during diastole as the aortic valve closes, and deflates at isovolumic contraction. The hemodynamic effects of IABP counterpulsation pertain largely to changes in afterload and coronary perfusion. Inflation of the balloon during diastole causes a volume displacement and augments the Windkessel effect, which in turn increases peripheral perfusion.[31] Because the intraaortic blood volume has been displaced during diastole, there is a reduction in intraaortic blood volume (and, in turn, pressure) during isovolumic contraction. This effect serves two purposes: first, it reduces the impedance against which the LV ejects and thus decreases afterload; second, it causes earlier opening of the aortic valve and reduces the time

spent in isovolumic contraction, in turn lowering myocardial oxygen demand. The reduced oxygen demand, together with an increase in DBP and in turn coronary perfusion pressure, improves the balance of myocardial oxygen supply and demand. IABP counterpulsation, through a decrease in the Effective arterial elastance (Ea) slope, leads to a modest increase in stroke volume in patients with available contractile reserve. Despite these many hemodynamic benefits, it is important to note that the IABP provides a form of pressure, but not volume unloading for the LV. This effect is shown by little to no leftward shift of the LVEDV on the PV loop (**Fig. 3**).

Practical Considerations

The device is typically inserted via the femoral artery, although the axillary artery may also be used. The balloon sits in the descending aorta distal to the left subclavian artery and proximal to the renal arteries and ideally should extend from the left subclavian artery to the celiac artery branch. Its diameter during inflation should be 90% to 95% of the diameter of the descending aorta.[29] Although 40-cc balloons are often used in adult patients, undersizing the balloon reduces the efficacy of counterpulsation, and oversizing increases the risk of vascular complications.

The IABP is particularly useful in patients with high systemic vascular resistance but with hypotension limiting the use of afterload-reducing medications. In these instances, counterpulsation decreases systemic vascular resistance without a significant decrease in systemic blood pressure. IABP can be particularly useful in patients with acute severe mitral regurgitation to support forward ejection of blood into the aorta.

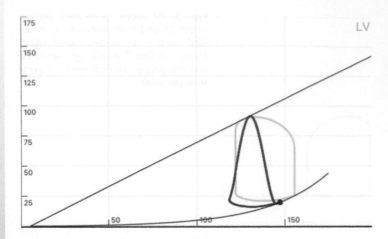

Fig. 4. PV loops generated during acute CS and Impella. Green loop = CS. Red loop = Impella. Developed using Harvi - online.[34] x-axis represents LV volume (ml); y-axis represents LV pressure (mmHg).

TRANSAORTIC MICROAXIAL FLOW PUMP (IMPELLA)

The Impella devices (Abiomed, Danvers, MA, USA) are percutaneous transvalvular microaxial flow pumps. The impeller is fixed to a pigtail catheter, which is advanced across the aortic valve into the LV. The impeller draws blood from the LV and ejects it into the proximal aorta. The flow achieved depends on the head pressure (the differential pressure between the aorta and LV) and the speed of the motor pump.

Hemodynamic Effects

These devices are continuous flow pumps; thus, blood is continuously ejected from the LV to the aorta independent of the phase of the cardiac cycle, providing circulatory support and resulting in several hemodynamic changes (**Fig. 4**). First, the continuous drainage of blood from the LV causes a decrease in preload and afterload as it exerts both a volume and pressure unloading effect on the ventricle. This effect results in a leftward and downward shift of the PV loop. Second, the shape of the PV loop changes from its normal trapezoidal shape to a more triangular shape, reflecting loss of the energy-consuming phases of isovolumic contraction and relaxation. The combination of the leftward shift and change in PV loop shape reduces myocardial oxygen demand. There may also be a modest increase in coronary perfusion pressure with a decrease in LVEDP and a direct increase in total cardiac output.

Practical Considerations

Three models are presently used in practice for left-sided support, with the model number reflecting the maximal flow rate that can be achieved: Impella 2.5, Impella CP (3.5), and Impella 5.0. The femoral artery is typically used for insertion, although the axillary artery may also be used, particularly if ambulation is required or if there is concern that the patient may require femoral-femoral venoarterial extracorporeal membrane oxygenation (VA-ECMO).

LEFT ATRIUM TO AORTA FLOW PUMP (TandemHeart)

The TandemHeart (CardiacAssist Inc, Pittsburgh, PA, USA) is a percutaneously inserted extracorporeal centrifugal flow pump. It indirectly unloads volume from the LV via direct left atrial unloading and provides circulatory support by pumping blood into the femoral artery.

Hemodynamic Effects

Similar to the Impella device, the TandemHeart system decreases preload albeit through indirect LV unloading. However, in contrast to the Impella system, the retrograde blood flow support from femoral artery to the aorta pressurizes the arterial system and increases afterload. This effect can be seen by a leftward, but not downward shift of the PV loop (**Fig. 5**). Therefore, the TandemHeart provides LV volume unloading without LV pressure unloading.

Practical Considerations

The TandemHeart system is percutaneously placed with a 21F venous inflow cannula inserted in the femoral vein and 17F cannula in the femoral artery. The venous inflow cannula extends up to the right atrium and crosses the septum (via Brockenbrough atrial transseptal puncture technique) into the left atrium (LA). Blood is directly drained from the LA, passes through a continuous-flow, extracorporeal centrifugal pump, and is

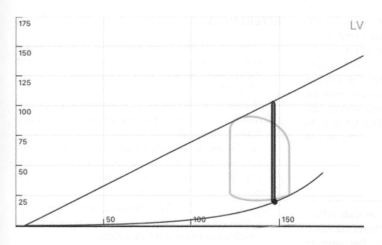

Fig. 5. PV loops generated during acute CS and TandemHeart. Green loop = CS. Red loop = TandemHeart. Developed using Harvi - online.[34] x-axis represents LV volume (ml); y-axis represents LV pressure (mmHg).

ejected into the outflow cannula, which typically ends in the iliac artery.

VENOARTERIAL EXTRACORPOREAL MEMBRANE OXYGENATION

VA-ECMO provides extracorporeal MCS and simultaneous gas exchange for acute cardiorespiratory failure.[32] VA-ECMO can be established via central or peripheral access. This section focuses on peripheral cannulation because this is typically used for refractory CS and cardiac arrest outside of the operating room. Peripheral VA-ECMO is often initiated via femoral artery and femoral or internal jugular vein access. There are, however, other configurations for VA-ECMO that provide unique advantages and challenges.[33]

Hemodynamic Effects

Femoral-femoral VA-ECMO provides excellent circulatory support with flows of 3 to 4 L/min typically used. In addition, drainage of blood from the right atrium decreases right ventricular preload and peripheral venous congestion. However, despite draining blood from the right heart, VA-ECMO may not decrease LV preload because of the residual pulmonary blood flow, Thebesian drainage of coronary blood flow, aortic regurgitation (if present), and return of bronchial blood flow to the left atrium. In order for the blood that enters the LV to be ejected, the native LV must generate enough pressure to overcome the increased afterload created by the retrograde ECMO flow support. An inability for the LV to perform this task will result in LV distention resulting in an increase in both LVEDP and wall stress. Therefore, peripheral VA-ECMO may cause an *increase* in LV preload and afterload, especially at higher ECMO flow rates (**Fig. 6**).

LV venting strategies may be used in order to reduce LV preload and afterload. There are at least 8 different strategies for LV unloading with VA-ECMO that include simply reducing ECMO flow rates, starting inotropic medications, adding

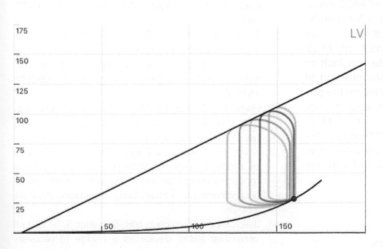

Fig. 6. PV loops generated during acute CS and peripheral VA-ECMO with an unvented LV. Green loop = CS. Pink loop = ECMO flow at 2 L/min. Blue loop = ECMO flow at 3 L/min. Purple loop = ECMO flow at 4 L/min. Yellow loop = ECMO flow at 4.75 L/min. Developed using Harvi - online.[34] x-axis represents LV volume (ml); y-axis represents LV pressure (mmHg).

surgical or percutaneous direct LV venting cannulas/catheters as well as other MCS devices in conjunction with VA-ECMO. The use of an Impella with VA-ECMO (termed "ECPELLA") is physiologically beneficial in theory because it provides direct LV decompression, decreases pulmonary venous congestion, and provides additional antegrade flow support into the aortic root. The latter acts to decrease blood stasis and mitigates the risk of aortic root thrombosis.

Practical Considerations

Peripheral VA-ECMO comprises a venous inflow cannula, pump, oxygenator, and arterial cannula. In a femoral-femoral configuration, the venous cannula drains blood from the superior vena cava, right atrium, and inferior vena cava via the femoral vein. The deoxygenated blood then passes through the pump and oxygenator and is returned as oxygenated blood via a femoral arterial cannula that ends in the iliac artery or distal portion of the descending aorta. Venous cannulas are typically 19F to 25F, whereas arterial cannulas are often 15F to 24F. A 6F to 8F vascular introducer is also placed distal to the arterial cannula to provide antegrade femoral blood flow to the leg and prevent ischemic injury.

SUMMARY

The incidence of CS is increasing; however, its prognosis remains dismal despite revascularization therapies. Major advances in MCS device design have led to several possible platforms that can be used for patients with CS. These potential therapies are reflected by an increase in the utilization of MCS over the past decade.[30] However, there is currently a paucity of data to determine patient selection, timing of MCS initiation, as well as the optimal MCS device for specific clinical scenarios. As a result, there is likely a wide variation regarding the management of MCS among different institutions. Despite this lack of standardization, it is crucial that determination of the optimal MCS device for CS is based on the patient's unique hemodynamic profile, and the hemodynamic characteristics of the specific MCS device. It is through the translation of these underlying physiologic principles that one can attempt to maximize the clinical utility of MCS and improve outcomes in CS.

DISCLOSURE

The authors have nothing to disclose.

REFERENCES

1. Thiele H, Zeymer U, Neumann F-J, et al. Intraaortic balloon support for myocardial infarction with cardiogenic shock. N Engl J Med 2012;367: 1287–96.
2. Reynolds HR, Hochman JS. Cardiogenic shock: current concepts and improving outcomes. Circulation 2008;117:686–97.
3. van Diepen S, Katz JN, Albert NM, et al. Contemporary management of cardiogenic shock: a scientific statement from the American Heart Association. Circulation 2017;136:e232–68.
4. Mandawat A, Rao SV. Percutaneous mechanical circulatory support devices in cardiogenic shock. Circ Cardiovasc Interv 2017;10:e004337.
5. Puymirat E, Fagon JY, Aegerter P, et al. Cardiogenic shock in intensive care units: evolution of prevalence, patient profile, management and outcomes, 1997-2012. Eur J Heart Fail 2017;19:192–200.
6. Babaev A, Frederick PD, Pasta DJ, et al. Trends in management and outcomes of patients with acute myocardial infarction complicated by cardiogenic shock. JAMA 2005;294:448–54.
7. Goldberg RJ, Spencer FA, Gore JM, et al. Thirty-year trends (1975-2005) in the magnitude of, management of, and hospital death rates associated with cardiogenic shock in patients with acute myocardial infarction: a population-based perspective. Circulation 2009;119:1211.
8. Kolte D, Khera S, Aronow WS, et al. Trends in incidence, management, and outcomes of cardiogenic shock complicating ST-elevation myocardial infarction in the United States. J Am Heart Assoc 2014; 3:e000590.
9. Jeger RV, Radovanovic D, Hunziker PR, et al. Ten-year trends in the incidence and treatment of cardiogenic shock. Ann Intern Med 2008;149: 618–26.
10. Uriel N, Sayer G, Annamalai S, et al. Mechanical unloading in heart failure. J Am Coll Cardiol 2018;72: 569–80.
11. Cohn JN, Goldstein SO, Greenberg BH, et al. A dose-dependent increase in mortality with vesnarinone among patients with severe heart failure. Vesnarinone Trial Investigators. N Engl J Med 1998;339: 1810–6.
12. Hajjar LA, Teboul J-L. Mechanical circulatory support devices for cardiogenic shock: state of the art. Crit Care 2019;23:76.
13. Kormos RL, Cowger J, Pagani FD, et al. The Society of Thoracic Surgeons Intermacs database annual report: evolving indications, outcomes, and scientific partnerships. J Heart Lung Transplant 2019;38: 114–26.
14. Jakovljevic DG, Yacoub MH, Schueler S, et al. Left ventricular assist device as a bridge to recovery

for patients with advanced heart failure. J Am Coll Cardiol 2017;69:1924–33.

15. Rihal CS, Naidu SS, Givertz MM, et al. 2015 SCAI/ACC/HFSA/STS Clinical Expert Consensus Statement on the Use of Percutaneous Mechanical Circulatory Support Devices in Cardiovascular Care: endorsed by the American Heart Association, the Cardiological Society of India, and Sociedad Latino America. J Am Coll Cardiol 2015;65:e7–26.

16. Ponikowski P, Voors AA, Anker SD, et al. 2016 ESC Guidelines for the diagnosis and treatment of acute and chronic heart failure: the Task Force for the diagnosis and treatment of acute and chronic heart failure of the European Society of Cardiology (ESC). Developed with the special contribution of the Heart Failure Association (HFA) of the ESC. Eur J Heart Fail 2016;18:891–975.

17. Lindenfeld J, Albert NM, Boehmer JP, et al. HFSA 2010 Comprehensive Heart Failure Practice Guideline. J Card Fail 2010;16:e1–194.

18. Burkhoff D, Sayer G, Doshi D, et al. Hemodynamics of mechanical circulatory support. J Am Coll Cardiol 2015;66:2663–74.

19. Kapur NK, Esposito M. Hemodynamic support with percutaneous devices in patients with heart failure. Heart Fail Clin 2015;11:215–30.

20. Stulak JM, Davis ME, Haglund N, et al. Adverse events in contemporary continuous-flow left ventricular assist devices: a multi-institutional comparison shows significant differences. J Thorac Cardiovasc Surg 2016;151:177–89.

21. Long B, Robertson J, Koyfman A, et al. Left ventricular assist devices and their complications: a review for emergency clinicians. Am J Emerg Med 2019;37:1562–70.

22. Harvey L, Holley C, Roy SS, et al. Stroke after left ventricular assist device implantation: outcomes in the continuous-flow era. Ann Thorac Surg 2015;100:535–41.

23. Leuck A-M. Left ventricular assist device driveline infections: recent advances and future goals. J Thorac Dis 2015;7:2151–7.

24. Hieda M, Sata M, Seguchi O, et al. Importance of early appropriate intervention including antibiotics and wound care for device-related infection in patients with left ventricular assist device. Transplant Proc 2014;46:907–10.

25. Kapur NK, Paruchuri V, Jagannathan A, et al. Mechanical circulatory support for right ventricular failure. JACC Heart Fail 2013;1:127–34.

26. Argiriou M, Kolokotron S-M, Sakellaridis T, et al. Right heart failure post left ventricular assist device implantation. J Thorac Dis 2014;6(Suppl 1):S52–9.

27. Kushnir VM, Sharma S, Ewald GA, et al. Evaluation of GI bleeding after implantation of left ventricular assist device. Gastrointest Endosc 2012;75:973–9.

28. Gilotra NA, Stevens GR. Temporary mechanical circulatory support: a review of the options, indications, and outcomes. Clin Med Insights Cardiol 2014;8:75–85.

29. Parissis H, Graham V, Lampridis S, et al. IABP: history-evolution-pathophysiology-indications: what we need to know. J Cardiothorac Surg 2016;11:122.

30. Stretch R, Sauer CM, Yuh DD, et al. National trends in the utilization of short-term mechanical circulatory support: incidence, outcomes, and cost analysis. J Am Coll Cardiol 2014;64:1407–15.

31. Bonios MJ, Pierrakos CN, Argiriou M, et al. Increase in coronary blood flow by intra-aortic balloon counterpulsation in a porcine model of myocardial reperfusion. Int J Cardiol 2010;138:253–60.

32. Rao P, Khalpey Z, Smith R, et al. Venoarterial extracorporeal membrane oxygenation for cardiogenic shock and cardiac arrest. Circ Heart Fail 2018;11:e004905.

33. Rao P, Alouidor B, Smith R, et al. Ambulatory central VA-ECMO with biventricular decompression for acute cardiogenic shock. Catheter Cardiovasc Interv 2017. https://doi.org/10.1002/ccd.27428.

34. Burkhoff D, Dickstein M, Schleicher T. Harvi - Online. Available at: http://harvi.online. Accessed April 14, 2020.

Cardiac Emergencies in Patients with Left Ventricular Assist Devices

Jay D. Pal, MD, PhD, Joseph Cleveland, MD, Brett T. Reece, MD,
Jessica Byrd, RN, Christopher N. Pierce, MS, CCP, Andreas Brieke, MD,
William K. Cornwell III, MD*

KEYWORDS

- Blood pressure • Continuous-flow left ventricular assist device • Cardiogenic shock

KEY POINTS

- Continuous-flow left ventricular assist devices are frequently used for management of patients with advanced heart failure with reduced ejection fraction.
- Although technologic advancements have contributed to improved outcomes, several complications arise over time.
- These complications result from several factors, including medication effects, physiologic responses to chronic exposure to circulatory support that is minimally/entirely nonpulsatile, and dysfunction of the device itself.
- Clinical presentation can range from chronic and indolent to acute, life-threatening emergencies.
- Several areas of uncertainty exist regarding best practices for managing complications; however, growing awareness has led to development of new guidelines to reduce risk and improve outcomes.

INTRODUCTION

Continuous-flow left ventricular assist devices (CF-LVADs) are an increasingly used strategy for management of patients with advanced heart failure with reduced ejection fraction (HFrEF).[1,2] Although these devices are associated with significant improvements in quality of life[3] and survival,[4–6] CF-LVAD implantation is associated with several adverse events, including stroke,[7] nonsurgical bleeding,[8] pump thrombosis,[4,9] right ventricular (RV) dysfunction, and progressive heart failure.[10,11] A host of physiologic (mal)adaptations result from chronic exposure to continuous-flow

circulatory support. Specifically, sympathetic nerve activity is markedly increased as a result of baroreceptor unloading, which predisposes to hypertension and possibly stroke.[7,12–14] In addition, shearing forces applied to blood and plasma products as they traverse through the device lead to an acquired von Willebrand syndrome, which increases the risk of bleeding.[15] Medications considered standard of care, specifically anticoagulants and antihypertensive agents, may complicate management as well. The pump itself is composed of multiple internal and external components, which must function appropriately in

Sources of Funding: Dr W.K. Cornwell has received funding by an NIH/NHLBI Mentored Patient-Oriented Research Career Development Award (#1K23HLI32048-01), as well as the NIH/NCATS (#UL1TR002535), Susie and Kurt Lochmiller Distinguished Heart Transplant Fund, the Clinical Translational Science Institute at the University of Colorado Anschutz Medical Campus, and Medtronic Inc. Dr J.D. Pal has received funding from Medtronic Inc.

Department of Medicine-Cardiology, University of Colorado Anschutz Medical Campus, 12631 East 17th Avenue, B130, Office 7107, Aurora, CO 80045, USA

* Corresponding author. 12631 East 17th Avenue, B130, Office 7107, Aurora, CO 80045.

E-mail address: william.cornwell@cuanschutz.edu

Heart Failure Clin 16 (2020) 295–303
https://doi.org/10.1016/j.hfc.2020.02.003
1551-7136/20/© 2020 Elsevier Inc. All rights reserved.

order to provide adequate hemodynamic support for the patient. Malfunction of any one of these parts may threaten the well-being of the patient and in severe cases, may also lead to an LVAD emergency.

All of these factors work together in an almost synergistic fashion to increase the risk of major adverse events, characterized by hemodynamic instability with end-organ damage and in some cases, overt emergencies. Depending on the nature and severity of the LVAD emergency, some complications may be managed medically, whereas others may require emergent surgical consultation for definitive therapy.

LEFT VENTRICULAR ASSIST DEVICES: DEVICE DESIGN AND STRUCTURE

Current-generation CF-LVADs have a common basic structure composed of both internal and external components. The HeartMate II CF-LVAD is an "axial" flow pump, which contains an inflow cannula that is surgically connected to the LV apex. The newer HeartWare HVAD and HeartMate III LVADs, also continuous-flow pumps, are "centrifugal" flow devices, which are much smaller, intrapericardial pumps and are directly connected to the heart. Each type of CF-LVAD has a rotating impeller that propels oxygenated blood forward through an outflow cannula, which is surgically anastomosed to the arterial circulation, typically the ascending aorta. The devices require a continuous source of power in order to function. The power supply is provided by a percutaneous lead that exits the skin, typically in either the left or right upper abdominal quadrant, and connects the internal pump to an external power source. The power source may come from either alternating current (AC), such as a power unit connected to a wall socket, or direct current (DC), such as batteries that the patient straps to his/her person.

ASSESSING PERFUSION IN PATIENTS WITH CONTINUOUS-FLOW LEFT VENTRICULAR ASSIST DEVICE

CF-LVAD patients may or may not have detectable pulses peripherally, depending on the amount of pulsatility generated throughout the cardiac cycle. CF-LVAD flow is directly proportional to pump speed and inversely proportional to pressure differential across the pump, determined by[16,17]:

Pressure differential = outflow (aortic) pressure - inflow (left ventricular) pressure

For this reason, pulsatility varies throughout the cardiac cycle and is typically greatest during systole, when LV pressure increases and the pressure differential across the pump declines. During diastole, LV pressure declines, the pressure differential across the pump increases, and consequently, CF-LVAD flow declines. In situations where there is no meaningful systolic phase of the cardiac cycle, such as ventricular fibrillation or cardiogenic shock, flow may be entirely nonpulsatile and the patient will not have a detectable pulse on clinical examination. Otherwise, these patients typically have some degree of pulsatility, albeit a nonphysiologic and markedly diminished pulse pressure compared with normal individuals.

Given the unique characteristics of flow among CF-LVAD patients, alternative methods of assessing adequacy of systemic perfusion may be necessary in cases of clinical instability. The lack of a physiologic pulse may render standard blood pressure (BP) assessments by automated oscillometric cuff, sphygmomanometer, or noninvasive BP, unreliable, and the inability to detect a pulse using any of these methods does not necessarily suggest that perfusion is inadequate. As such, either arterial catheter, or manual BP assessment with Doppler is recommended to determine whether perfusion is sufficient.[18] Waveform capnography, which was incorporated into the 2015 American Heart Association (AHA) guidelines for cardiopulmonary resuscitation,[19] is an additional method of determining adequacy of perfusion in unconscious CF-LVAD patients. Because peak end-tidal carbon dioxide level (P_{ETCO2}) reflects adequacy of systemic perfusion in the setting of cardiogenic shock, a P_{ETCO2} level less than 20 mm Hg, in an intubated and unconscious CF-LVAD patient, indicates that flow is insufficient and chest compressions are necessary. Alternatively, a higher P_{ETCO2} level in an unconscious, intubated patient suggests that perfusion is adequate and noncardiac factors account for the instability.[18]

The authors' center has developed protocols for evaluation of CF-LVAD patients experiencing acute medical problems (**Fig. 1**). For patients who are alert and responsive, a physical examination and device interrogation are completed. For patients who are stable, the patient is evaluated for common device complications such as stroke, infection, or RV dysfunction. For unstable patients, the patient is urgently evaluated for complications such as ventricular arrhythmias (VA), sepsis, bleeding, or device malfunction and managed appropriately.

The authors' protocol for management of the unresponsive CF-LVAD patient is displayed in the event that perfusion is inadequate, external chest compressions may be necessary, particularly in cases where the CF-LVAD is not

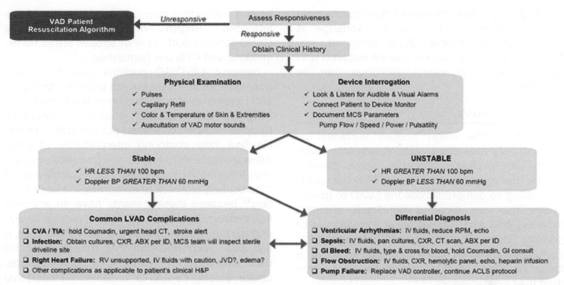

Fig. 1. University of Colorado Hospital algorithm for assessment of the CF-LVAD patient with an acute medical problem.

functioning appropriately or is off. Following initiation of external chest compressions, we recommend following local emergency medical services (EMS) and advanced cardiovascular life support (ACLS) protocols. They also also recommend that regional LVAD centers partner with local EMS facilities, particularly in areas where CF-LVAD patients are known to reside, so that emergency crews are familiarized with the unique aspects of managing these patients.

DEVICE-RELATED EMERGENCIES
Electrical Failure of the Pump

The Achilles heel of modern CF-LVADs remains the percutaneous driveline. The driveline carries power to the device, and all available pumps have redundancy built into the driveline to prevent catastrophic failures. The individual wires in the driveline are separately shielded and the entire driveline is encased in a protective casing. However, with increasing durations of support, the repetitive flexing of the driveline can result in disruption of the shielding. This can lead to a short-to-shield phenomenon, which occurs when the current from one phase in the driveline is shorted to the driveline shielding, which is grounded. This results in intermittent pump stoppages when connected to AC power. The immediate treatment is to return the patient to battery power and/or use an ungrounded cable to the system monitor.[20] A phase short is less common but occurs when a short-circuit occurs within 2 wires within the driveline. This can also result in intermittent pump

stoppages and cannot be resolved by using battery power or an ungrounded cable. The clinical challenge is identifying the underlying problem, but the intermittent nature of the pump stoppages makes diagnosis difficult. Detailed log file analysis can identify the underlying electrical problem, but this type of analysis is not immediately available.[21] The authors recommend that all patients with suspected electrical failure be admitted for log file analysis and provocative testing to identify the underlying problem in an environment where pump stoppages can be managed expeditiously.

The damaged portion of the driveline can be external and diagnosed by physical examination and radiographic examination. Radiography or computed tomography scanning can demonstrate the internal wires of the driveline and any potential areas of disruption. The intracorporeal portion of the driveline can similarly be evaluated radiographically. In the event of external damage, the driveline can be repaired by individually splicing each internal wire to a new driveline. This is an effective therapy and can be performed reliably.[22] If the driveline damage is intracorporeal, the only available therapy is surgical pump exchange.

Less frequent, but more emergent, is severe trauma to the driveline that results in transection or disruption of multiple leads within the driveline, causing pump stoppage. In the case of significant damage to the driveline, the LVAD cannot be restarted, and the appropriate treatment depends on the patient's clinical status. In patients who are hemodynamically stable, driveline repair can be performed as discussed earlier. If driveline repair is not possible, and the patient is an appropriate surgical candidate, then pump exchange is reasonable. For unstable patients, temporary mechanical circulatory support may be required until driveline repair or pump exchange can be performed.

Pump Thrombosis

Because of the blood contact surfaces, all commercially available LVADs require anticoagulation with warfarin.[23] Although some patients can be managed with lower levels of anticoagulation, doing so can predispose the LVAD to thrombosis. This has received significant attention recently, and avoiding thrombus formation is of primary importance in patient management.[9] Fortunately, current generation pumps have a lower incidence of de novo thrombus formation than their predecessors.[24–26]

Diagnosis of pump thrombosis can be made by changes in power consumption, markers of hemolysis, and decreased clinical effect of mechanical support.[27,28] In reasonable surgical candidates, pump exchange is the most effective treatment available. However, patients who present with pump thrombosis are at higher risk for developing subsequent thrombus, and therefore, anticoagulation management must be modified in this scenario. Exchange of a second-generation LVAD (eg, HeartMate II) to a third-generation pump (eg, HeartWare HVAD, HeartMate III) has been shown to be effective, although the evidence is limited to small case series. Furthermore, this technique requires a more involved operation than simply replacing the pump body. Subcostal exchange techniques are safe and effective and can be used for a variety of LVADs.[29–32]

For patients deemed not candidates for surgical exchange, numerous groups have reported on the use of thrombolytics.[33] Unfortunately, this therapy is only occasionally effective, and the risk of recurrent thrombosis is high.[34,35] Furthermore, the risk of bleeding complications precludes the use of this therapy in many patients. The HeartWare HVAD seems more amenable to lytic therapy than the HeartMate II.[34,36]

COMMON MEDICAL EMERGENCIES AMONG PATIENTS WITH CONTINUOUS-FLOW LEFT VENTRICULAR ASSIST DEVICE
Acute Stroke

The rate of strokes among CF-LVAD patients is unacceptably high.[7] Approximately 10% of individuals suffer from a stroke in the first year of support alone, and between 6 and 24 months of support, stroke is the primary cause of death among this patient population.[1] According to the Interagency Registry for Mechanically Assisted Circulatory Support, 51% of strokes are ischemic in cause and 49% are hemorrhagic.[37]

Because CF-LVAD patients cannot undergo brain MRI, clinical assessment is limited to history and physical examination, computed tomography imaging, and vascular studies. Transcranial Doppler may be considered but the lack of pulsatile flow may confound interpretation of data. Although ischemic strokes are frequently treated with thrombolytics, CF-LVAD patients may be at a particularly high risk of hemorrhagic transformation[38] because these patients have an acquired von Willebrand syndrome and also receive aspirin and warfarin as per standard of care.[23] As such, it has been recommended that thrombolytics be used cautiously for treatment of acute ischemic stroke among CF-LVAD patients.[38] Intraarterial endovascular therapy may be considered as well. In a single-center experience of 5 CF-LVAD patients with middle cerebral artery syndrome who underwent mechanical thrombectomy, vessel recanalization was successful in all cases.[39]

Management of hemorrhagic strokes can be problematic in these patients. Generally, management of intracerebral hemorrhagic involves correcting the coagulopathy and BP control.[40] Reversal agents such as vitamin K, prothrombin complex, or fresh frozen plasma will reduce risk of hemorrhage expansion, while simultaneously increasing risk of formation of a CF-LVAD pump thrombus. For that reason, partial versus full reversal of international normalized ratio (INR) levels may be considered on a case-by-case basis. CF-LVAD patients are predisposed to chronic hypertension for several reasons, including baroreceptor-mediated increases in sympathetic tone[7,12,14] and heightened diastolic BP in the setting of continuous flow.[7] As such, these patients are not uncommonly on several classes of antihypertensive agents and/or *goal-directed medical therapy* to maintain a normal mean arterial pressure (MAP). It is recommended that MAP be maintained at 80 mm Hg or less to reduce risk of stroke among stable outpatients.[23,41] In the setting of acute hemorrhagic stroke, aggressive antihypertensive management may be necessary to reduce MAP to target levels.

Gastrointestinal Bleeding

Gastrointestinal (GI) bleeding is one of the most common complications associated with CF-LVADs and affects almost one-third of patients in the first year of support alone.[6] Several mechanisms account for this bleeding risk, including therapeutic anticoagulation, acquired von

Willebrand syndrome, and development of arteriovenous malformations resulting from a nonphysiologic pulse.[42,43] For those individuals who suffer from recurrent GI bleeding, adjustments to their medication regimen are made, such as a reduction or discontinuation of their antiplatelet agent, reduction in INR target, and possibly the addition of agents such as octreotide[42] or danazol.[44] In addition, there is evidence to suggest that digoxin may reduce the rate of GI bleeding through inhibition of hypoxia-inducible factor 1-alpha.[45]

The presentation of GI bleeding ranges from occult bleeding to life-threatening hemorrhage. Severe cases require emergent consultation with gastroenterologists with endoscopy to identify and treat the location of the bleed, as well as blood transfusions as clinically indicated. The severity of GI bleeds among CF-LVAD patients tends to be worse than the general population, on average necessitating 2 to 4 units of packed red blood cell transfusions.[46] However, blood transfusions increase the amount of circulating antibodies in the bloodstream and consequently, may make it difficult to match organs for CF-LVAD patients who are supported as a bridge-to-transplantation strategy.

Ventricular Arrhythmias

VA are common following CF-LVAD implantation and affect up to 20% to 50% of patients.[47–51] Individuals with a history of ischemic and nonischemic cardiomyopathies seem to be at similar risk, regardless of whether VA were present before device implantation.[49,52–55] Mechanisms of VA include ischemia and fibrosis, mechanical disruption of the myocardium resulting from the inflow cannula, and electrophysiological remodeling (shortening of the QRS duration and lengthening of the QTc).[54,56,57] The clinical presentation of VA is highly variable. Many individuals have minimal or no symptoms, and arrhythmias are incidentally detected by electrocardiography.[58,59] However, it is well recognized that VA may precipitate RV dysfunction, which may in turn lead to cardiogenic shock due to a reduction in LV preload.[51,53,56,60,61]

Medical management of VA among CF-LVAD patients consists primarily of amiodarone and/or sodium channel blocking antiarrhythmic agents such as lidocaine or procainamide.[56] Catheter ablation procedures may be necessary for refractory arrhythmias, with a short-term success rate of approximately 80%.[56,62,63]

Aortic Insufficiency

Aortic insufficiency leading to hemodynamic compromise is usually a chronic process, but patients can present acutely when the regurgitant volume exceeds the ability of the device to mobilize the increased preload.[64] Subsequently, the left ventricular pressures and volumes increase, leading to pulmonary edema and RV dysfunction. In some patients, increasing pump speed may temporarily alleviate symptoms, but in those with relatively high afterload, this may exacerbate the problem by decreasing LV pressures and increasing the regurgitant fraction.

No optimal treatment of aortic insufficiency in patients supported with CF-LVADs exists, as all available therapies have significant limitations. Surgical aortic valve replacement (or aortic valve closure) carries significant risk of reoperative cardiac surgery in patients who are typically in a decompensated state and poor surgical candidates. In appropriate patients, however, surgical AVR is most likely to result in complete resolution of aortic insufficiency.[65,66]

Percutaneous closure of the aortic valve with an Amplatzer septal occluder has also been reported, with favorable results such as immediate improvement in hemodynamics and reduction in left-sided filling pressures.[67,68] However, some patients will develop hemolysis because the occluder does allow for some high-velocity regurgitant jets to remain. In patients in whom the regurgitation is completely abolished, the hemolysis resolves. This therapy is appropriate for patients who are poor surgical candidates, although long-term results of this intervention are unknown.

More recently, transcatheter aortic valve replacement has been used to treat for LVAD-associated aortic insufficiency.[69] Unfortunately, most are case reports or small case series.[70,71] Challenges to this therapy result from the noncalcified nature of the aortic annulus, which limits stability and positioning of the prosthesis. We have obtained good results with a combination of a Corevalve (Medtronic, Minneapolis, MN) and Sapien3 (Edwards Lifesciences, Irvine, CA), but this technique incurs significant procedural cost. By using the Corevalve as a scaffold in the native root, the Sapien3 balloon-expandable valve is secure and eliminates a perivalvular leak. Others have reported using valve prostheses with good results.[72] Although procedural success rates are high, overall survival remains limited, likely reflecting the morbid nature of this condition.

Cardiac Arrest

Guidelines for basic life support (BLS) and advanced cardiovascular life support (ACLS) among normal individuals define a cardiac arrest based on the presence or absence of a pulse.[73] As previously noted, CF-LVAD patients may not have detectable pulses, which may make it difficult to determine whether a patient requires these therapies in settings of hemodynamic instability.[74] In one single-center experience, the decision to initiate BLS/ACLS for unstable CF-LVAD patients was significantly delayed compared with controls without CF-LVADs.[74] This delay was due, at least in part, to implementation of different techniques to assess adequacy of perfusion, such as digital palpation of a pulse, Doppler assessment of BP, or measurement of MAP with an arterial catheter, as well as determination of CF-LVAD flow on the device programmer. Because of these issues, in 2017 the AHA released an official statement on cardiopulmonary resuscitation for individuals supported by mechanical circulatory support devices.[18]

The 2 most common reasons for failure of the device are loss of power and driveline failure.[18] Therefore, the clinical assessment of an unstable CF-LVAD patient should include an evaluation of pump function to verify that the device has a sufficient supply of power, whether it is from AC (power wall unit) or DC (batteries) power supply. CF-LVAD drivelines, although durable and designed with built-in redundancy, are nevertheless at risk of damage from wear and tear over time, kinking, fracture, and partial/complete severing. Driveline compromise associated with device malfunction will typically initiate alarms from the device, which may indicate that power to the device has been compromised. However, alarms are only present when the pump has a power source and attempts to restart the device have failed. Compressions are recommended for CF-LVAD patients, when clinical instability is determined to be cardiac in cause.[18]

SUMMARY

CF-LVADs are a life-saving strategy for patients with advanced HFrEF and significantly improve quality of life. However, there are several adverse events associated with current-generation devices that limit improvements in outcome that these patients might otherwise enjoy. These adverse events result from several factors, including medication effects, physiologic responses to a reduction in pulsatility, shearing forces imposed on blood and plasma products, and pump dysfunction. These factors may work together in an almost synergistic fashion to create an environment that predisposes patients to medical and surgical emergencies. Although recommendations for management of some of these complications are lacking, there is a growing awareness and interest in improving outcomes for these patients, which has led to the recent development of guidelines

and safeguards to reduce and prevent the rate of emergencies in this population.

DISCLOSURE

Dr J.D. Pal has received research funding from Medtronic Inc and is a consultant for Medtronic Inc. Dr. Cornwell has received research funding from Medtronic Inc and is a consultant for Medtronic Inc. Mr C.N. Pierce is a consultant for Abbott. The other authors have nothing to disclose.

REFERENCES

1. Kirklin JK, Pagani FD, Kormos RL, et al. Eighth annual INTERMACS report: special focus on framing the impact of adverse events. J HeartLung Transplant 2017;36(10):1080–6.
2. Yancy CW, Jessup M, Bozkurt B, et al. 2013 ACCF/AHA guideline for the management of heart failure: a report of the American College of Cardiology Foundation/American Heart Association Task Force on Practice Guidelines. Circulation 2013;128: e240–327.
3. Rogers JG, Aaronson KD, Boyle AJ, et al. Continuous flow left ventricular assist device improves functional capacity and quality of life of advanced heart failure patients. J Am CollCardiol 2010; 55(17):1826–34.
4. Rogers JG, Pagani FD, Tatooles AJ, et al. Intrapericardial left ventricular assist device for advanced heart failure. NEngl J Med 2017;376(5):451–60.
5. Mehra MR, Goldstein DJ, Uriel N, et al. Two-year outcomes with a magnetically levitated cardiac pump in heart failure. NEngl J Med 2018;378(15):1386–95.
6. Estep JD, Starling RC, Horstmanshof DA, et al. Risk assessment and comparative effectiveness of left ventricular assist device and medical management in ambulatory heart failure patients: results from the ROADMAP study. J Am CollCardiol 2015; 66(16):1747–61.
7. Cornwell WK III, Ambardekar AV, Tran T, et al. Stroke incidence and impact of continuous-flow left ventricular assist devices on cerebrovascular physiology. Stroke 2019;50:542–8.
8. Wever-Pinzon O, Selzman CH, Drakos SG, et al. Pulsatility and the risk of nonsurgical bleeding in patients supported with the continuous-flow left ventricular assist device HeartMate II. CircHeart Fail 2013;6(3):517–26.
9. Starling RC, Moazami N, Silvestry SC, et al. Unexpected abrupt increase in left ventricular assist device thrombosis. NEngl J Med 2014;370(1):33–40.
10. Hayek S, Sims DB, Markham DW, et al. Assessment of right ventricular function in left ventricular assist

device candidates. CircCardiovascImaging 2014; 7(2):379–89.

11. Lampert BC, Teuteberg JJ. Right ventricular failure after left ventricular assist devices. J HeartLung Transplant 2015;34(9):1123–30.

12. Cornwell WK 3rd, Tarumi T, Stickford A, et al. Restoration of pulsatile flow reduces sympathetic nerve activity among individuals with continuous-flow left ventricular assist devices. Circulation 2015; 132(24):2316–22.

13. Cornwell WK 3rd, Tarumi T, Aengevaeren VL, et al. Effect of pulsatile and nonpulsatile flow on cerebral perfusion in patients with left ventricular assist devices. J HeartLung Transplant 2014;33(12): 1295–303.

14. Markham DW, Fu Q, Palmer MD, et al. Sympathetic neural and hemodynamic responses to upright tilt in patients with pulsatile and nonpulsatile left ventricular assist devices. CircHeart Fail 2013;6(2): 293–9.

15. Uriel N, Pak SW, Jorde UP, et al. Acquired von Willebrand syndrome after continuous-flow mechanical device support contributes to a high prevalence of bleeding during long-term support and at the time of transplantation. J Am CollCardiol 2010;56(15): 1207–13.

16. Pagani FD. Continuous-flow rotary left ventricular assist devices with "3rd generation" design. SeminThoracCardiovasc Surg 2008;20(3):255–63.

17. Moazami N, Fukamachi K, Kobayashi M, et al. Axial and centrifugal continuous-flow rotary pumps: a translation from pump mechanics to clinical practice. J HeartLung Transplant 2013;32(1):1–11.

18. Peberdy MA, Gluck JA, Ornato JP, et al. Cardiopulmonary resuscitation in adults and children with mechanical circulatory support: a scientific statement from the American Heart Association. Circulation 2017;135(24):e1115–34.

19. Link MS, Berkow LC, Kudenchuk PJ, et al. Part 7: adult advanced cardiovascular life support: 2015 American Heart Association guidelines update for cardiopulmonary resuscitation and emergency cardiovascular care. Circulation 2015;132(18 Suppl 2): S444–64.

20. Coyle L, Graney N, Gallagher C, et al. Treatment of HeartMate II short-to-shield patients with an ungrounded cable: indications and long-term outcomes. ASAIO J 2019 Apr 18. https://doi.org/10.1097/MAT.0000000000001012.

21. Flint KM, Brieke A, Cornwell WK 3rd, et al. HeartMate II system controller failure presenting as driveline fault with repeated pump stoppages. CircHeart Fail 2019;12(7):e005738.

22. Stulak JM, Schettle S, Haglund N, et al. Percutaneous driveline fracture after implantation of the HeartMate II left ventricular assist device: how durable is driveline repair? ASAIO J 2017;63(5):542–5.

23. Slaughter MS, Pagani FD, Rogers JG, et al. Clinical management of continuous-flow left ventricular assist devices in advanced heart failure. J HeartLung Transplant 2010;29(4 Suppl):S1–39.

24. McGee E Jr, Danter M, Strueber M, et al. Evaluation of a lateral thoracotomy implant approach for a centrifugal-flow left ventricular assist device: The LATERAL clinical trial. J HeartLung Transplant 2019;38(4):344–51.

25. Mehra MR, Naka Y, Uriel N, et al. A fully magnetically levitated circulatory pump for advanced heart failure. N Engl J Med 2017;376(5):440–50.

26. Uriel N, Colombo PC, Cleveland JC, et al. Hemocompatibility-related outcomes in the MOMENTUM 3 trial at 6 months: a randomized controlled study of a fully magnetically levitated pump in advanced heart failure. Circulation 2017;135(21):2003–12.

27. Uriel N, Morrison KA, Garan AR, et al. Development of a novel echocardiography ramp test for speed optimization and diagnosis of device thrombosis in continuous-flow left ventricular assist devices: the Columbia ramp study. J Am CollCardiol 2012; 60(18):1764–75.

28. Jorde UP, Aaronson KD, Najjar SS, et al. Identification and management of pump thrombus in the HeartWareleft ventricular assist device system: a novel approach using log file analysis. JACCHeart Fail 2015;3(11):849–56.

29. Gaffey AC, Chen CW, Chung JJ, et al. Improved approach with subcostal exchange of the HeartMate II left ventricular assist device: difference in on and off pump? Ann Thorac Surg 2017;104(5): 1540–6.

30. Soleimani B, Stephenson ER, Price LC, et al. Clinical experience with sternotomy versus subcostal approach for exchange of HeartMate II left ventricular assist device. Ann Thorac Surg 2015;100(5): 1577–80.

31. Ota T, Yerebakan H, Akashi H, et al. Continuous-flow left ventricular assist device exchange: clinical outcomes. J HeartLung Transplant 2014;33(1):65–70.

32. Agarwal R, Kyvernitakis A, Soleimani B, et al. Clinical experience of HeartMate II to HeartWareleft ventricular assist device exchange: a multicenter experience. Ann Thorac Surg 2019;108(4):1178–82.

33. Schlendorf K, Patel CB, Gehrig T, et al. Thrombolytic therapy for thrombosis of continuous flow ventricular assist devices. J Card Fail 2014;20(2):91–7.

34. Upshaw JN, Kiernan MS, Morine KJ, et al. Incidence, management, and outcome of suspected continuous-flow left ventricular assist device thrombosis. ASAIO J 2016;62(1):33–9.

35. Dang G, Epperla N, Muppidi V, et al. Medical management of pump-related thrombosis in patients with continuous-flow left ventricular assist devices: a systematic review and meta-analysis. ASAIO J 2017;63(4):373–85.

36. Saeed D, Maxhera B, Albert A, et al. Conservative approaches for HeartWare ventricular assist device pump thrombosis may improve the outcome compared with immediate surgical approaches. InteractCardiovascThorac Surg 2016; 23(1):90–5.

37. Acharya D, Loyaga-Rendon R, Morgan CJ, et al. INTERMACSanalysis of stroke during support with continuous-flow left ventricular assist devices: risk factors and outcomes. JACCHeart Fail 2017;5(10): 703–11.

38. Willey JZ, Demmer RT, Takayama H, et al. Cerebrovascular disease in the era of left ventricular assist devices with continuous flow: risk factors, diagnosis, and treatment. J HeartLung Transplant 2014;33(9): 878–87.

39. Rice CJ, Cho SM, Zhang LQ, et al. The management of acute ischemic strokes and the prevalence of large vessel occlusion in left ventricular assist device. Cerebrovasc Dis 2018;46(5–6):213–7.

40. Hemphill JC 3rd, Greenberg SM, Anderson CS, et al. Guidelines for the management of spontaneous intracerebral hemorrhage: a guideline for healthcare professionals from the American Heart Association/American Stroke Association. Stroke 2015;46(7):2032–60.

41. Lampert BC, Eckert C, Weaver S, et al. Blood pressure control in continuous flow left ventricular assist devices: efficacy and impact on adverse events. Ann Thorac Surg 2014;97(1):139–46.

42. Molina TL, Krisl JC, Donahue KR, et al. Gastrointestinalbleeding in left ventricular assist device: octreotide and other treatment modalities. ASAIO J 2018; 64(4):433–9.

43. Kang J, Hennessy-Strahs S, Kwiatkowski P, et al. Continuous-flow LVADsupport causes a distinct form of intestinal angiodysplasia. Circ Res 2017; 121(8):963–9.

44. Schettle S, Bawardy BA, Asleh R, et al. Danazol treatment of gastrointestinal bleeding in left ventricular assist device-supported patients. J HeartLung Transplant 2018;37(8):1035–7.

45. Vukelic S, Vlismas PP, Patel SR, et al. Digoxin is associated with a decreased incidence of angiodysplasia-related gastrointestinal bleeding in patients with continuous-flow left ventricular assist devices. CircHeartFail 2018;11(8):e004899.

46. Birks EJ. Stopping LVADbleeding: a piece of the puzzle. Circ Res 2017;121(8):902–4.

47. Raasch H, Jensen BC, Chang PP, et al. Epidemiology, management, and outcomes of sustained ventricular arrhythmias after continuous-flow left ventricular assist device implantation. Am Heart J 2012;164(3):373–8.

48. Nakahara S, Chien C, Gelow J, et al. Ventricular arrhythmias after left ventricular assist device. CircArrhythmElectrophysiol 2013;6(3):648–54.

49. Bedi M, Kormos R, Winowich S, et al. Ventricular arrhythmias during left ventricular assist device support. Am J Cardiol 2007;99(8):1151–3.

50. Garan AR, Yuzefpolskaya M, Colombo PC, et al. Ventricular arrhythmias and implantable cardioverter-defibrillator therapy in patients with continuous-flow left ventricular assist devices: need for primary prevention? J Am CollCardiol 2013;61(25):2542–50.

51. Andersen M, Videbaek R, Boesgaard S, et al. Incidence of ventricular arrhythmias in patients on long-term support with a continuous-flow assist device (HeartMate II). J HeartLung Transplant 2009; 28(7):733–5.

52. Slaughter MS, Rogers JG, Milano CA, et al. Advanced heart failure treated with continuous-flow left ventricular assist device. NEngl J Med 2009; 361(23):2241–51.

53. Ziv O, Dizon J, Thosani A, et al. Effects of left ventricular assist device therapy on ventricular arrhythmias. J Am CollCardiol 2005;45(9): 1428–34.

54. Harding JD, Piacentino V, Rothman S, et al. Prolonged repolarization after ventricular assist device support is associated with arrhythmias in humans with congestive heart failure. J Card Fail 2005; 11(3):227–32.

55. Oswald H, Schultz-Wildelau C, Gardiwal A, et al. Implantable defibrillator therapy for ventricular tachyarrhythmia in left ventricular assist device patients. Eur J Heart Fail 2010;12(6):593–9.

56. Gopinathannair R, Cornwell WK, Dukes JW, et al. Device therapy and arrhythmia management in left ventricular assist device recipients: a scientific statement from the American Heart Association. Circulation 2019;139(20):e967–89.

57. Harding JD, Piacentino V 3rd, Gaughan JP, et al. Electrophysiological alterations after mechanical circulatory support in patients with advanced cardiac failure. Circulation 2001;104:1241–7.

58. Oz MC, Rose EA, Slater J, et al. Malignant ventricular arrhythmias are well tolerated in patients receiving long-term left ventricular assist devices. J Am CollCardiol 1994;24(7):1688–91.

59. Sims DB, Rosner G, Uriel N, et al. Twelve hours of sustained ventricular fibrillation supported by a continuous-flow left ventricular assist device. Pacing ClinElectrophysiol 2012;35(5):e144–8.

60. Kadado AJ, Akar JG, Hummel JP. Arrhythmias after left ventricular assist device implantation: incidence and management. TrendsCardiovasc Med 2018; 28(1):41–50.

61. Cantillon DJ, Bianco C, Wazni OM, et al. Electrophysiologic characteristics and catheter ablation of ventricular tachyarrhythmias among patients with heart failure on ventricular assist device support. Heart rhythm 2012;9(6):859–64.

62. Sacher F, Reichlin T, Zado ES, et al. Characteristics of ventricular tachycardia ablation in patients with continuous flow left ventricular assist devices. CircArrhythmElectrophysiol 2015;8(3):592–7.

63. Dandamudi G, Ghumman WS, Das MK, et al. Endocardial catheter ablation of ventricular tachycardia in patients with ventricular assist devices. Heart Rhythm 2007;4(9):1165–9.

64. Truby LK, Garan AR, Givens RC, et al. Aortic insufficiency during contemporary left ventricular assist device support: analysis of the INTERMACSregistry. JACCHeart Fail 2018;6(11):951–60.

65. Schechter MA, Joseph JT, Krishnamoorthy A, et al. Efficacy and durability of central oversewing for treatment of aortic insufficiency in patients with continuous-flow left ventricular assist devices. J HeartLung Transplant 2014;33(9):937–42.

66. Atkins BZ, Hashmi ZA, Ganapathi AM, et al. Surgical correction of aortic valve insufficiency after left ventricular assist device implantation. J ThoracCardiovasc Surg 2013;146(5):1247–52.

67. Grohmann J, Blanke P, Benk C, et al. Trans-catheter closure of the native aortic valve with an Amplatzer-Occluder to treat progressive aortic regurgitation after implantation of a left-ventricular assist device. Eur J Cardiothorac Surg 2011;39(6):3.

68. Parikh KS, Mehrotra AK, Russo MJ, et al. Percutaneous transcatheter aortic valve closure successfully treats left ventricular assist device-associated aortic insufficiency and improves cardiac hemodynamics. JACCCardiovascInterv 2013;6(1):84–9.

69. Pal JD, McCabe JM, Dardas T, et al. Transcatheter aortic valve repair for management of aortic insufficiency in patients supported with left ventricular assist devices. J Card Surg 2016;31(10):654–7.

70. Phan QT, Kim SW, Nguyen HL. Percutaneous closure of congenital Gerbode defect using Nit-Occlud((R)) Le VSD coil. World J Cardiol 2017; 9(7):634–9.

71. Rene AG, Desai N, Wald J, et al. Transfemoraltranscatheter aortic valve replacement with a self-expanding valve for severe aortic regurgitation in a patient with left ventricular assist device. J Card Surg 2017;32(11):741–5.

72. Yehya A, Rajagopal V, Meduri C, et al. Short-term results with transcatheter aortic valve replacement for treatment of left ventricular assist device patients with symptomatic aortic insufficiency. J HeartLung Transplant 2019;38(9):920–6.

73. Berg RA, Hemphill R, Abella BS, et al. Part 5: adult basic life support: 2010 American Heart Association guidelines for cardiopulmonary resuscitation and emergency cardiovascular care. Circulation 2010; 122(18 Suppl 3):S685–705.

74. Garg S, Ayers CR, Fitzsimmons C, et al. In-hospital cardiopulmonary arrests in patients with left ventricular assist devices. J Card Fail 2014;20(12): 899–904.

Acute Aortic Syndromes
Diagnostic and Therapeutic Pathways

Eduardo Bossone, MD, PhD, FCCP, FESC, FACC[a],[*],[1], Brigida Ranieri, PhD[b],[1], Luigia Romano, MD[c], Valentina Russo, MD[d], Luigi Barbuto, MD[c], Rosangela Cocchia, MD[a], Filomena Pezzullo, MD[c], Chiara Amato[e],[2], Olga Vriz, MD[f], Luigi Di Tommaso, MD[g], Gabriele Iannelli, MD[g], Martin Czerny, MD, MBA, FESC, MEBCTS, FEBVS[h]

KEYWORDS

- Acute aortic syndromes • Aortic dissection • Intramural hematoma • Penetrating aortic ulcer
- Multiparametric diagnostic algorithm • Surgical repair • Thoracic endovascular aortic repair

KEY POINTS

- Acute aortic syndromes are life-threatening medical conditions that include classic acute aortic dissection (AAD), aortic intramural hematoma, and penetrating aortic ulcer, as well as aortic pseudoaneurysm and traumatic aortic injury.
- The European Society of Cardiology aortic diseases guidelines provide a multiparametric diagnostic algorithm (clinical, laboratory, and imaging findings) to provide rapid and accurate stepwise diagnosis.
- Urgent surgical repair is recommended for type A AAD.
- The recommended management for uncomplicated type B AAD is aggressive medical therapy. In contrast, thoracic endovascular aortic repair is recommended for complicated type B AAD.
- AAD should be considered a lifelong disease that affects the entire aorta (holistic concept), requiring close clinical and imaging surveillance.

INTRODUCTION

Acute aortic syndromes (AASs) are life-threatening medical conditions sharing similar clinical characteristics and leading to a breakdown of the intima and media. They include classic acute aortic dissection (AAD), aortic intramural hematoma (IMH), and penetrating aortic ulcer (PAU), as well as aortic pseudoaneurysm and traumatic aortic injury.[1],[2] Given the nonspecific symptoms and physical signs, the diagnosis of AAS requires a high index of clinical suspicion promptly followed by an imaging test and related appropriate

Funding: This research did not receive any specific grant from funding agencies in the public, commercial, or not-for-profit sectors.

[a] Cardiology Division, Antonio Cardarelli Hospital, Via A. Cardarelli 9, Naples I-80131, Italy; [b] IRCCS SDN, Via Gianturco 113, Naples I-80142, Italy; [c] Department of General and Emergency Radiology, Antonio Cardarelli Hospital, Via Cardarelli 9, Naples I-80131, Italy; [d] Department of Advanced Biomedical Sciences, Federico II University of Naples, Via Pansini 5, Naples I-80131, Italy; [e] Faculty of Medicine, Federico II University of Naples, Via Pansini 5, Naples I-80131, Italy; [f] Echocardiography Department, Heart Centre, King Faisal Specialist Hospital & Research Centre, MBC-16, PO Box 3354, Riyadh 11211, Saudi Arabia; [g] Cardiac Surgery Division, Department of Advanced Biomedical Sciences, Federico II University of Naples, Via Pansini 5, Naples I-80131, Italy; [h] Department of Cardiovascular Surgery, Faculty of Medicine, University Heart Center Freiburg, Albert-Ludwigs-University of Freiburg, Breisacher Str. 86, Freiburg 79110, Germany

[1] These authors contributed equally.
[2] Present address: Via San Giacomo dei Capri 156, Naples I-80131, Italy.
* Corresponding author.
E-mail address: eduardo.bossone@aocardarelli.it

therapeutic interventions. This article discusses the current AASs diagnostic and therapeutic pathways.

CLASSIFICATION

AASs are commonly classified based on anatomic location of the lesion.[3] According to the Stanford classification, type A AAD (corresponding with DeBakey types I and II) involves the ascending aorta, irrespective of where the dissection began (**Fig. 1**), whereas type B dissection (corresponding with DeBakey type III) does not involve the ascending aorta (**Fig. 2**). Recently, the term non-A-non-B aortic dissection was introduced into current literature and into recommendations.[4] As to the fundamentally different natural course of the disease process, any affection of the aortic arch, either by the location of the primary entry tear at the level of the aortic arch or by retrograde extension of an IMH into the aortic arch from a primary type B aortic dissection, should be classified as non-A-non-B aortic dissection (**Fig. 3**). Based on the time from symptom onset to diagnosis, AASs are defined as acute (<14 days), subacute (15–90 days), or chronic (>90 days).[2]

A Deeper Look into Details

Recently, a new classification system for AAD has been proposed: the TEM (type, entry site,

malperfusion) system. The idea is in analogy to the tumor, node, metastasis (TNM) staging system in oncology, where here type refers to either type A, type B, or type non-A-non-B aortic dissection; entry site refers to E0 (no entry visible), E1 (entry located in the aortic root or ascending aorta), E2 (entry located within the aortic arch), or E3 (entry located in the descending aorta); and malperfusion is M0 (no malperfusion), M1 (malperfusion affecting the coronary arteries), M2 (malperfusion affecting the supraaortic vessels), or M3 (malperfusion affecting visceral, renal, and/or lower extremity branch vessels) with a further categorization as M– irrespective of the segment involved for patients without clinical signs of malperfusion but with true lumen collapse, and M+ for patients with additional clinical signs of malperfusion in the segment involved (**Fig. 4**).[5]

As an example, patients presenting with a type A AAD with a primary entry tear in the ascending aorta and no radiological or clinical signs of malperfusion are classified as type A, E1, M0, and ascending aortic replacement is the therapy of choice. Another example is a retrograde type A AAD with a primary entry tear distal to the left subclavian artery with a true lumen collapse at computed tomography angiography (CTA) at the level of the visceral and renal arteries with severe abdominal pain. Such patients are classified as type A, E3, M1+ and should undergo immediate

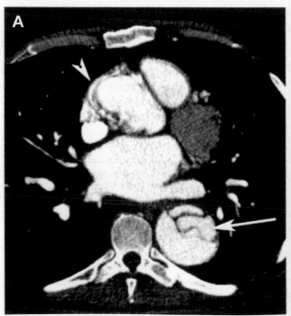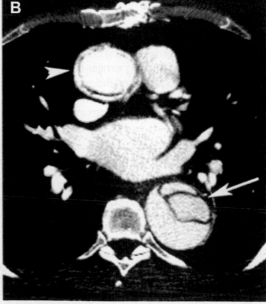

Fig. 1. Axial postcontrast computed tomography (CT) in a patient with type A AAD. Axial postcontrast CT images (A and B) showing irregularity of the aortic wall with an intimal flap between the true and false aortic lumens. There is compression of the true lumen of the ascending aorta (*white arrowheads, A and B*) and of the descending aorta (*white arrows, A and B*) by expanding false lumen. (*Courtesy of* the Department of General and Emergency Radiology, A. Cardarelli Hospital, Naples, Italy).

A

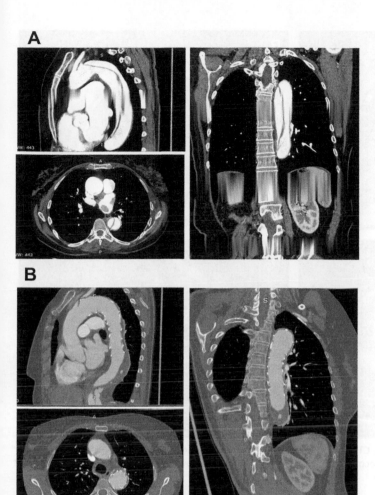

B

ascending and aortic arch replacement using the frozen elephant trunk (FET) technique to exclude the primary entry tear from circulation, which is highly likely to resolve visceral and renal malperfusion.

This new classification system is designed to provide deeper insights into the underlying pathophysiologic process, helping to define the extent of aortic repair, and allowing clinicians to obtain an initial prediction of perioperative outcome.

CLASSIC ACUTE AORTIC DISSECTION

AAD is characterized by the presence of an intimal flap separating the true lumen and the false lumen (FL).[2] The estimated incidence ranges between 2.6 and 3.5 cases per 100,000 person-years. It affects men more than women, particularly those in their fifth and sixth decades.[1,2,6]

Risk Factors

Most common risk factors for AAD are conditions associated with increased wall stress, such as hypertension (65%–75% of cases), atherosclerosis (27% of cases), and aortic aneurysm. In contrast, conditions associated with aortic media abnormalities consist of genetic disease (eg, Marfan syndrome or Loeys-Dietz syndrome, which are more frequent in young patients with AAD [<40 years]), vascular inflammation (eg, autoimmune disorders or infection), and deceleration trauma.[1,2,7] It is worth noting that iatrogenic type A AAD may also occur during heart catheterization, but it usually has a favorable outcome with conservative medical treatment.[8]

Clinical Features

Patients with AAD typically present with symptoms of abrupt onset of ripping, migratory chest and/or

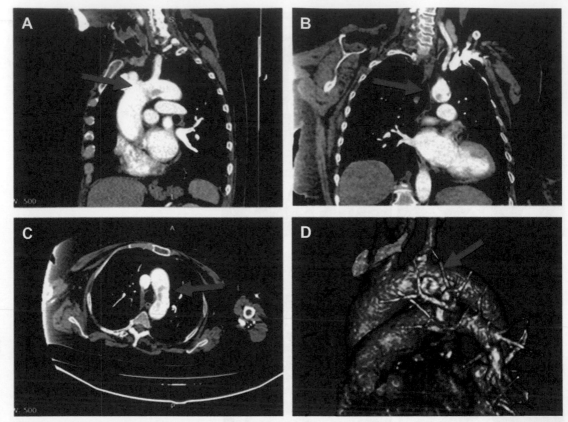

Fig. 3. Preoperative contrast-enhanced CT scan of localized aortic arch dissection (*arrows*). (*A–C*) Multiplanar reconstruction; (*D*) three-dimensional reconstruction. (*Courtesy of* the Cardiac Surgery Department, Federico II Medical School University, Naples, Italy).

back pain. In most cases, pain radiates to the anterior chest or neck when the ascending aorta is involved, and to the back when the descending thoracic aorta is involved. It should be highlighted that 6% of patients with AAD present with no pain.[2,7,9,10]

Complications may differ between patients with type A and type B AAD. In type A AAD, aortic regurgitation (40%–75%), cardiac tamponade (<20%), pleural effusion (15%), syncope (15%), myocardial ischemia or infarction (10%–15%), heart failure (<10%), major neurologic deficit (coma/stroke <10%), acute renal failure (<20%), lower limb ischemia (<10%), mesenteric ischemia (<5%), and spinal cord injury (<1%) are more frequent. In contrast, in type B AAD, lower rates

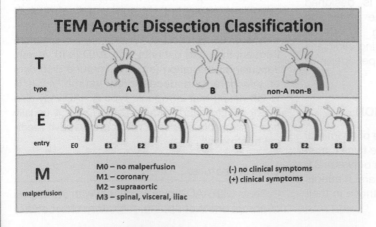

Fig. 4. TEM aortic dissection classification based on dissection extension, primary entry site, and end-organ malperfusion according to aortic segmentation. (*From* Sievers HH, Rylski B, Czerny M, et al. Aortic dissection reconsidered: type, entry site, malperfusion classification adding clarity and enabling outcome prediction [published online ahead of print, 2019 Nov 22]. Interact Cardiovasc Thorac Surg 2019;ivz281. https://doi.org/10.1093/icvts/ivz281; with permission.)

of acute renal failure (10%), heart failure (<5%), syncope (<5%), and major neurologic deficit (coma/stroke <5%) have been observed. Lower limb ischemia occurs with similar frequency (10%), whereas pleural effusion is more common (20%).[2]

Electrocardiogram and Chest Radiograph

Electrocardiograms (ECGs) and chest radiographs are of limited diagnostic value. More common ECG findings are nonspecific ST-T wave changes and left ventricular hypertrophy related to long-standing hypertension. Signs of myocardial ischemia/infarction may also be present in cases of coronary involvement. However, ECG may be within normal limits in more than 30% of patients.[11] Chest radiograph may reveal abnormal aortic contour and/or widening of the mediastinal silhouette. There may be evidence of pleural effusion and/or congestive heart failure. A normal-appearing chest radiograph is seen in more than 10% of documented cases of AAD.[11]

Laboratory Testing

Laboratory testing remains essential in the workup of patients with AAD. It may detect and/or confirm ongoing deadly complications, including myocardial infarction (troponin I or T), renal failure (creatinine), liver ischemia (aspartate transaminase/alanine aminotransferase), and bowel ischemia (lactate). In particular, D-dimer (a fibrin degradation product) levels proved to have high sensitivity for the diagnosis of AAD. A cutoff level of 500 ng/mL has been shown to rule out both pulmonary embolism and classic AAD within the first hours of symptom onset (sensitivity 95.7%, specificity 61.3%, negative predictive value 97.7% vs positive predictive value 45.2% at a cutoff level of 500 ng/mL within the first 6 hours).[12] However, D-dimer may be within normal limits in cases of thrombosed FL, IMH, and PAU.

Imaging Studies

Imaging techniques are a key step to confirm a clinically suspected AAS. The most frequently used technique is computed tomography (CT) followed by transthoracic echocardiography (TTE)/transesophageal echocardiography (TEE) and magnetic resonance imaging (MRI).[6,11] Data from the International Registry of Acute Aortic Dissection (IRAD) have shown that the use of CT has increased over the years as the initial diagnostic imaging modality in patients with type A AAD, from 46% to 73% (P<.001). In contrast, the use of TEE has decreased from 50% to 23%.[11] Patient clinical status (ie, hemodynamic stability), local availability, and expertise influence the choice of the most appropriate imaging modality.[2] Each approach presents advantages and limitations (**Table 1**).[2,6,13]

Echocardiography

TTE is usually the first imaging test performed among patients presenting to the emergency

Table 1
Relative strengths of imaging modalities for acute aortic syndromes

	TTE	TEE	MRI	CT
Imaging Factors				
Comprehensive aortic assessment	+	+ +	+ + +	+ + +
Tomographic (3D reconstruction)	−	−	+ + +	+ + +
Functional data	+ + +	+ + +	+ +	+
Tissue characterization	−	−	+ + +	+ + +
Clinical Factors				
Portability	+ + +	+ + +	−	−
Patient access/monitoring	+ + +	+ + +	+	+ +
Rapidity	+ + +	+ +	+ +	+ + +
Need for contrast media	−	−	+ +	+ + +
Need for sedation	−	+ + +	−	−
Lack of radiation exposure	+ + +	+ + +	+ + +	−
Serial examinations	+ +	+	+ + +	+ + (+)[a]

Plus (+) denotes a positive remark and minus (−) denotes a negative remark. The number of signs indicates the estimated potential value.

Abbreviations: 3D, three-dimensional; CT, computed tomography; MRI, magnetic resonance imaging; TEE, transesophageal echocardiography; TTE, transthoracic echocardiography

[a] +++only for follow-up after aortic stenting (metallic struts), otherwise limit radiation.

Modified from Bossone E, Suzuki T, Eagle KA, et al. Diagnosis of acute aortic syndromes: imaging and beyond. Herz. 2013;38(3):269–76.

room with chest pain. It has high accuracy in the detection of dissection involving the ascending aorta (sensitivity 77%–80%, specificity 93%–96%),[2] whereas sensitivity for type B AAD is low (31%–55%). It is therefore necessary to perform an additional imaging test to obtain a comprehensive aorta evaluation and to confirm or exclude AAD.

TEE (sensitivity 99%, specificity 89%) provides a comprehensive assessment of the aorta from its root to the descending aorta except for the distal ascending aorta (just before the innominate artery), which is not well visualized owing to the interposition of the right bronchus and trachea (blind spot). In addition, it does not permit assessment of the abdominal aorta. However, TEE should be considered a semi-invasive technique requiring sedation.[14] Furthermore, it cannot be performed in patients affected by esophageal diseases. TTE along with TEE may detect major complications such as pericardial effusion, aortic regurgitation, cardiac tamponade, and wall motion abnormalities, strongly affecting prognosis.[2,15]

Computed Tomography
CT (pooled sensitivity 100%, pooled specificity 98%), widely available and easily accessible, has an excellent spatial resolution allowing a comprehensive assessment of the entire aorta and its branch vessels. In addition, it may detect major complications.[2] ECG-gated acquisitions substantially reduce the occurrence of motion artifacts, avoiding potential pitfalls in AAS diagnosis. There is growing evidence that, in clinically uncomplicated type B AAD, the presence on initial CT of high-risk radiological features (primary entry tear diameter >10 mm; initial total aortic diameter ≥40 mm; FL diameter ≥22 mm; patent FL; partially thrombosed FL) may guide the patient toward a preemptive endovascular treatment instead of medical therapy alone.[16] Furthermore, in the emergency scenario, a triple rule-out CT strategy has been proposed for differential diagnosis among AAD, pulmonary embolism, and acute coronary syndrome. The burden of ionizing radiation limits CT use for serial follow-up, especially in young patients and women. In addition, iodinated contrast agents are contraindicated in patients with renal insufficiency and may trigger adverse allergic reactions.

Magnetic Resonance Imaging
MRI (sensitivity and specificity up to 98%, high spatial resolution)[2,17] provides detailed information about aortic anatomy and function. It is also useful for the detection of pericardial effusion, aortic regurgitation, and carotid artery dissection.[18] However, it remains less suitable in the emergency scenario (not widely available) because of long acquisition time and lack of patient compliance. Furthermore, MRI cannot be performed in patients with metal implants. In contrast, being ionizing radiation free, it is particularly indicated in young patients and for imaging surveillance during follow-up.

Aortography
Because of its invasive nature, retrograde aortography has now been replaced by noninvasive imaging techniques.

A Multiparametric Diagnostic Algorithm
The European Society of Cardiology aortic diseases guidelines present a multiparametric diagnostic algorithm (clinical features, D-dimer, and imaging findings) in order to provide rapid and accurate stepwise diagnosis. First, patients with suspected AAD should undergo a comprehensive clinical evaluation (medical history and physical examination). In this regard, it is advised to apply the clinical risk scoring system proposed in the 2010 American Heart Association (AHA)/American College of Cardiology (ACC) guidelines for the diagnosis and management of patients with thoracic aortic disease to assess the pretest clinical probability of AAD (low score 0–1 vs high score 2–3). Notably, when calculated at presentation, this score has a sensitivity of 95.7% in identifying AAD[2,19] (**Fig. 5**A). The complete diagnostic algorithm along with related steps is shown in **Fig. 5**B.

MANAGEMENT AND OUTCOME
Initial Medical Therapy

All patients with AAD, regardless of definitive treatment, should receive aggressive medical therapy to control blood pressure and heart rate.[6] Heart rate should be maintained at or less than 60 beats/min (bpm), and blood pressure should be kept as low as possible while allowing perfusion of the brain, kidneys, and other vital organs. Pain control with morphine sulfate is also recommended to attenuate sympathetic-induced catecholamine release.

Management of Type A Acute Aortic Dissection

Urgent surgical repair is recommended for patients with type A AAD.[2] Data from the IRAD registry over 17 years have shown a significant increase of surgical management for type A AAD (from 79% to 90%; P<.001).[11] Furthermore, overall in-hospital mortality (from 31% to 22%; P<.001) and surgical mortality (25% to 18%; P = .003) have decreased

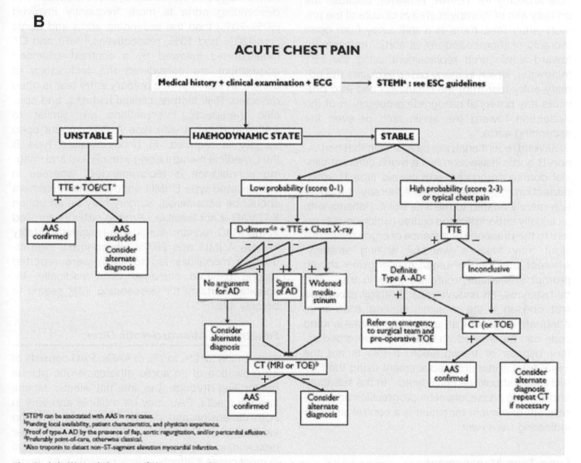

A

High-risk conditions	High-risk pain features	High-risk examination features
• Marfan syndrome (or other connective tissue diseases) • Family history of aortic disease • Known aortic valve disease • Known thoracic aortic aneurysm • Previous aortic manipulation (including cardiac surgery)	• Chest, back, or abdominal pain described as any of the following: - abrupt onset - severe intensity - ripping or tearing	• Evidence of perfusion deficit: - pulse deficit - systolic blood pressure difference - focal neurological deficit (in conjunction with pain) • Aortic diastolic murmur (new and with pain) • Hypotension or shock

B

Fig. 5. (A) Clinical data useful to assess the a priori probability of AAS. (B) Flowchart for decision making based on pretest sensitivity of AAS. AAS, acute aortic syndrome; AD, aortic dissection; CT, computed tomography; ECG, electrocardiogram; MRI, magnetic resonance imaging; STEMI, ST-elevation myocardial infarction; TOE, transesophageal echocardiography; TTE, transthoracic echocardiography. (*From* Erbel R, Aboyans V, Boileau C, et al. 2014 ESC guidelines on the diagnosis and treatment of aortic diseases: Document covering acute and chronic aortic diseases of the thoracic and abdominal aorta of the adult. The Task Force for the Diagnosis and Treatment of Aortic Diseases of the European Society of Cardiology (ESC). Eur Heart J 2014;35:2873-926; https://doi.org/10.1093/eurheartj/ehu281; with permission.)

significantly through the years.[11] In contrast, in-hospital mortality of patients treated with medical therapy alone has remained unacceptably high (57%; $P<.001$).[11] In particular, surgical repair was not performed in cases of coma, shock, malperfusion of coronary or peripheral arteries, and stroke.[11] It should be emphasized that old age (>70 years) per se should not be a reason for denying surgery.[20]

Management of Type B Acute Aortic Dissection

The recommended management for uncomplicated type B AAD is aggressive medical therapy to control blood pressure, heart rate, and pain, as described earlier (overall in-hospital mortality 13%, major deaths occurring within the first week).[2,11] In contrast, thoracic endovascular aortic repair (TEVAR) is currently recommended for complicated type B AAD.[2] In-hospital mortalities were significantly lower with endovascular treatment compared with open surgery (10.6% vs 33.9%; $P = .002$).[7,21] In-hospital mortalities of patients managed with TEVAR or medically were analogous (10.9% vs 8.7%; $P = .273$).[22] Open surgery may still be considered in cases of unfavorable anatomy for TEVAR. However, because the primary aim of therapy is always closure of the primary entry tear, there is a shift away from open thoracic or thoracoabdominal aortic replacement toward aortic arch replacement using the FET technique, which in many cases excludes the primary entry tear from the circulation and also prevents any potential retrograde propagation of the dissection toward the aortic arch or even the ascending aorta.[4]

Several recent analyses have shown that non-A-non-B aortic dissection has a much different clinical course compared with classic type B aortic dissection.[23,24] Patients require therapy, the question merely related to the time point. Patients with an initially uncomplicated course (which usually refers to the presence or absence of organ malperfusion) may have a watchful waiting strategy, whereas any kind of organ malperfusion should prompt immediate treatment. Also in these circumstances, an endovascular strategy should be first chosen if the proximal landing zone is of adequate length or if an adequate proximal landing zone can be created via subclavian-to-carotid artery bypass or transposition. If this is not the case, total aortic arch replacement using the FET technique should be considered.[4] In the subacute and chronic phase, diameter progression and subsequent aneurysm formation is a central issue for indicating treatment.

Long-Term Management

The 10-year survival rate has been reported to range between 30% and 60%.[6] In addition, a substantial delayed complication rate (progressive aortic insufficiency, aneurysm formation and rupture, recurrent dissection, leakage/hemorrhage at surgical anastomoses/stent-grafted sites) has been observed, especially during the first year from the index event. Thus, AAD should be considered a lifelong disease that affects the entire aorta (holistic concept), requiring close clinical and imaging surveillance (at discharge; 3, 6, 9, 12 months; and every year afterward). Medical treatment consists of blood pressure (<120 mm Hg) and heart rate (<60 bpm) control. Low-density lipoprotein cholesterol should be kept to less than 70 mg/dL (first choice: statins) classifying patients with AAD into the high-risk

category. Strict adherence to medical treatment should be monitored in these patients.

OTHER FORMS OF ACUTE AORTIC SYNDROMES
Intramural Hematoma

IMH accounts for 10% to 25% of AASs, caused by hemorrhage into the medial layer of the aorta.[2] The descending aorta is more frequently involved (60%–70%) than the ascending aorta and aortic arch (30% and 10%, respectively).[2] MRI and CT (unenhanced followed by a contrast-enhanced acquisition) are considered the techniques of choice. In this regard, a primary entry tear is often detected. Risk factors, clinical features, and specific therapeutic interventions are similar to AAD.[2] In patients with type A IMH, urgent open surgery is required. In uncomplicated type B IMH, medical therapy along with clinical and imaging surveillance is recommended, whereas in complicated type B IMH endovascular treatment should be considered. Surgery may be an option if TEVAR is not feasible.[2] Among patients enrolled in the IRAD registry, surgical in-hospital mortality in type A IMH was 26.6%. In contrast, high in-hospital mortalities (up to 40%) were reported among patients managed only medically. In-hospital mortality for descending IMH seems to be only 4%.[7,25]

Penetrating Atherosclerotic Ulcer

Accounting for 2% to 7% of AASs, PAU consists of an ulceration of an aortic atherosclerotic plaque penetrating through the internal elastic lamina into the media. PAU may be multiple and vary in both dimension and depth.[2] The most common location of PAU (>90%) is the middle and lower descending thoracic aorta (type B PAU),[26,27] and in most cases it affects elderly patients (>65 years) as a localized expression of systemic atherosclerosis. CTA is the diagnostic imaging technique of choice. Open surgery should be considered for ascending aorta PAU (type A). Medical therapy along with clinical and imaging surveillance is recommended for uncomplicated type B PAU, whereas endovascular treatment should be considered in complicated type B PAU. Open surgery remains an alternative in cases of contraindications to endovascular treatment.[2]

Traumatic Aortic Injury

Partial or complete transection of the aorta (90% of cases at the level of aortic isthmus) occurs as a result of major blunt thoracic trauma, frequently caused by a high-speed motor vehicle accident

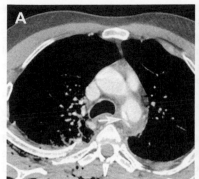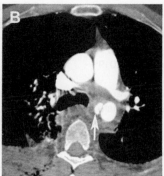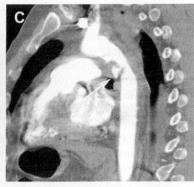

Fig. 6. Postcontrast CT of aortic traumatic injury. (*A*) Axial postcontrast CT image showing a posttraumatic aortic dissection at the level of the aortic isthmus. An intimal flap is present with aortic contour irregularity and extravasation of contrast medium (*white arrow*) associated with a mediastinal hematoma. (*B*) Axial postcontrast CT image showing a posttraumatic aortic pseudoaneurysm at the level of the aortic isthmus (*white arrow*) associated with a mediastinal hematoma. (*C*) Oblique sagittal postcontrast CT reconstruction showing a posttraumatic aortic pseudoaneurysm at the level of the aortic isthmus with contrast agent outpouching extending beyond the aortic wall (*white arrow*). (*Courtesy of* the Department of General and Emergency Radiology, A Cardarelli Hospital, Naples, Italy).

(**Fig. 6**). Most patients with complete aortic transection do not survive long enough for appropriate therapeutic interventions. CTA is also the imaging technique of choice for detecting other organ involvement (brain, visceral, and bone injury).[28–30] In the presence of favorable anatomy and local expertise, TEVAR should be preferred rather than surgery.

SUMMARY

AASs are life-threatening medical conditions including classic AAD, aortic IMH, and PAU, as well as aortic pseudoaneurysm and traumatic aortic injury. The European Society of Cardiology aortic diseases guidelines present a multiparametric diagnostic algorithm (clinical, laboratory, and imaging findings) to allow rapid and accurate stepwise diagnosis. All patients with AAD, regardless of definitive treatment, should receive aggressive medical therapy to control blood pressure and heart rate. Urgent surgical repair is recommended for type A AAD. The recommended management for uncomplicated type B AAD is aggressive medical therapy. In contrast, TEVAR is recommended for complicated type B. However, it remains a matter of debate whether and when TEVAR should be used in patients with uncomplicated type B AAD to prevent late complications. AAD should be considered a lifelong disease that affects the entire aorta (holistic concept), requiring close clinical and imaging surveillance.

DISCLOSURE

The authors have nothing to disclose.

REFERENCES

1. Hiratzka LF, Bakris GL, Beckman JA, et al. 2010 ACCF/AHA/AATS/ACR/ASA/SCA/SCAI/SIR/STS/ SVM Guidelines for the diagnosis and management of patients with Thoracic Aortic Disease: a report of the American College of Cardiology Foundation/ American Heart Association Task Force on Practice Guidelines, American Association for Thoracic Surgery, American College of Radiology, American Stroke Association, Society of Cardiovascular Anesthesiologists, Society for Cardiovascular Angiography and Interventions, Society of Interventional Radiology, Society of Thoracic Surgeons, and Society for Vascular Medicine. Circulation 2010;121: e266–369.

2. Erbel R, Aboyans V, Boileau C, et al, ESC Committee for Practice Guidelines. 2014 ESC Guidelines on the diagnosis and treatment of aortic diseases: Document covering acute and chronic aortic diseases of the thoracic and abdominal aorta of the adult. The Task Force for the Diagnosis and Treatment of Aortic Diseases of the European Society of Cardiology (ESC). Eur Heart J 2014;35: 2873–926.

3. Nienaber CA, Clough RE. Management of acute aortic dissection. Lancet 2015;385:800–11.

4. Czerny M, Schmidli J, Adler S, et al, EACTS/ESVS Scientific Document Group. Current options and recommendations for the treatment of thoracic aortic pathologies involving the aortic arch: an expert consensus document of the European Association for Cardio-Thoracic surgery (EACTS) and the European Society for Vascular Surgery (ESVS). Eur J Cardiothorac Surg 2019; 55:133–62.

5. Sievers HH, Rylski B, Czerny M, et al. Aortic dissection reconsidered: type, entry site, malperfusion classification adding clarity and enabling outcome prediction [published online ahead of print, 2019 Nov 22]. Interact Cardiovasc Thorac Surg 2019; ivz281. https://doi.org/10.1093/icvts/ivz281.

6. Bossone E, LaBounty TM, Eagle KA. Acute aortic syndromes: diagnosis and management, an update. Eur Heart J 2018;39:739–749d.

7. Evangelista A, Isselbacher EM, Bossone E, et al, IRAD Investigators. Insights from the International Registry of Acute Aortic Dissection: a 20-year experience of collaborative clinical research. Circulation 2018;137:1846–60.

8. Núñez-Gil IJ, Bautista D, Cerrato E, et al, Registry on Aortic Iatrogenic Dissection (RAID) Investigators. Incidence, management, and immediate- and long-term outcomes after iatrogenic aortic dissection during diagnostic or interventional coronary procedures. Circulation 2015;131:2114–9.

9. Hagan PG, Nienaber CA, Isselbacher EM, et al. The International Registry of Acute Aortic Dissection (IRAD): new insights into an old disease. JAMA 2000;283:897–903.

10. Park SW, Hutchison S, Mehta RH, et al. Association of painless acute aortic dissection with increased mortality. Mayo Clin Proc 2004;79:1252–7.

11. Pape LA, Awais M, Woznicki EM, et al. Presentation, diagnosis, and outcomes of acute aortic dissection: 17-year trends from the International Registry of Acute Aortic Dissection. J Am Coll Cardiol 2015; 66:350–8.

12. Suzuki T, Distante A, Zizza A, et al, IRAD-Bio Investigators. Diagnosis of acute aortic dissection by D-dimer: the International Registry of Acute Aortic Dissection Substudy on Biomarkers (IRAD-Bio) experience. Circulation 2009;119: 2702–7.

13. Baliga RR, Nienaber CA, Bossone E, et al. The role of imaging in aortic dissection and related syndromes. JACC Cardiovasc Imaging 2014;7: 406–24.

14. Goldstein SA, Evangelista A, Abbara S, et al. Multimodality imaging of diseases of the thoracic aorta in adults: from the American Society of Echocardiography and the European Association of Cardiovascular Imaging: endorsed by the Society of Cardiovascular Computed Tomography and Society for Cardiovascular Magnetic Resonance. J Am Soc Echocardiogr 2015;28:119–82.

15. Bossone E, Evangelista A, Isselbacher E, et al, International Registry of Acute Aortic Dissection Investigators. Prognostic role of transesophageal echocardiography in acute type A aortic dissection. Am Heart J 2007;153:1013–20.

16. Tadros RO, Tang GHL, Barnes HJ, et al. Optimal treatment of uncomplicated type B aortic dissection:

JACC review topic of the week. J Am Coll Cardiol 2019;74:1494–504.

17. Shiga T, Wajima Z, Apfel CC, et al. Diagnostic accuracy of transesophageal echocardiography, helical computed tomography, and magnetic resonance imaging for suspected thoracic aortic dissection: systematic review and meta-analysis. Arch Intern Med 2006;166:1350–6.

18. Nienaber CA, Kische S, Rousseau H, et al, INSTEAD-XL Trial. Endovascular repair of type B aortic dissection: long-term results of the randomized investigation of stent grafts in aortic dissection trial. Circ Cardiovasc Interv 2013;6: 407–16.

19. Rogers AM, Hermann LK, Booher AM, et al, IRAD Investigators. Sensitivity of the aortic dissection detection risk score, a novel guideline-based tool for identification of acute aortic dissection at initial presentation: results from the International Registry of Acute Aortic Dissection. Circulation 2011;123: 2213–8.

20. Trimarchi S, Eagle KA, Nienaber CA, et al, International Registry of Acute Aortic Dissection Investigators. Role of age in acute type A aortic dissection outcome: report from the International Registry of Acute Aortic Dissection (IRAD). J Thorac Cardiovasc Surg 2010;140:784–9.

21. Tsai TT, Isselbacher EM, Trimarchi S, et al, International Registry of Acute Aortic Dissection. Acute type B aortic dissection: does aortic arch involvement affect management and outcomes? Insights from the International Registry of Acute Aortic Dissection (IRAD). Circulation 2007;116(11 Suppl): I150–6.

22. Fattori R, Montgomery D, Lovato L, et al. Survival after endovascular therapy in patients with type B aortic dissection: a report from the International Registry of Acute Aortic Dissection (IRAD). JACC Cardiovasc Interv 2013;6:876–82.

23. Urbanski PP, Wagner M. Acute non-A-non-B aortic dissection: surgical or conservative approach? Eur J Cardiothorac Surg 2016;49:1249–54.

24. Rylski B, Pérez M, Beyersdorf F, et al. Acute non-A non-B aortic dissection: incidence, treatment and outcome. Eur J Cardiothorac Surg 2017;52:1111–7.

25. Harris KM, Braverman AC, Eagle KA, et al. Acute aortic intramural hematoma: an analysis from the International Registry of Acute Aortic Dissection. Circulation 2012;126(11 Suppl 1):S91–6.

26. Pate JW, Cole FH Jr, Walker WA, et al. Penetrating injuries of the aortic arch and its branches. Ann Thorac Surg 1993;55:586–92.

27. Jánosi RA, Gorla R, Tsagakis K, et al. Thoracic endovascular repair of complicated penetrating aortic ulcer: an 11-year single-center experience. J Endovasc Ther 2016;23:150–9.

28. Patel NH, Stephens KE Jr, Mirvis SE, et al. Imaging of acute thoracic aortic injury due to blunt trauma: a review. Radiology 1998;209:335–48.

29. Richens D, Kotidis K, Neale M, et al. Rupture of the aorta following road traffic accidents in the United Kingdom 1992-1999. The results of the co-operative crash injury study. Eur J Cardiothorac Surg 2003;23:143–8.

30. Azizzadeh A, Keyhani K, Miller CC 3rd, et al. Blunt traumatic aortic injury: initial experience with endovascular repair. J Vasc Surg 2009;49:1403–8.

Pulmonary Embolism
A Practical Guide for the Busy Clinician

Pablo Demelo-Rodriguez, MD, PhD[a,b,c], Francisco Galeano-Valle, MD[a,b,c], Andrea Salzano, MD[d], Eweline Biskup, MD[e,f], Olga Vriz, MD, PhD[g], Antonio Cittadini, MD[h], Lorenzo Falsetti, MD, PhD[i], Brigida Ranieri, PhD[d], Valentina Russo, MD[j], Anna Agnese Stanziola, MD, PhD[k,l], Eduardo Bossone, MD, PhD, FCCP, FESC, FACC[m], Alberto M. Marra, MD, PhD[h,n,*]

KEYWORDS

- Echocardiography • Biomarkers • Chronic thromboembolic pulmonary hypertension
- Deep venous thrombosis • Pulmonary embolism • Thrombolysis • Venous thromboembolism

KEY POINTS

- Acute pulmonary embolism (PE) is the third most common acute cardiovascular condition, and its prevalence tends to grow over time.
- Echocardiography is the most available, bedside, low-cost, diagnostic procedure for patients with PE.
- D-dimer has a very high negative predictive value, and if normal levels of D-dimer are detected, the diagnosis of PE is very unlikely.
- In case of persisting dyspnea during follow-up of a patient with PE, a transthoracic echocardiography should be performed in order to assess the risk of pulmonary hypertension.

This research did not receive any specific grant from funding agencies in the public, commercial, or not-for-profit sectors.

[a] Venous Thromboembolism Unit, Internal Medicine, Hospital General Universitario Gregorio Marañón, Calle doctor Esquerdo, 46, Madrid 28007, Spain; [b] Sanitary Research Institute Gregorio Marañón, Calle doctor Esquerdo, 46, Madrid 28007, Spain; [c] Universidad Complutense de Madrid, School of Medicine, Spain; [d] IRCCS SDN, Diagnostic and Nuclear Research Institute, Via Gianturco 131, Naples 80137, Italy; [e] Department of Basic Medical College, Shanghai University of Medicine and Health Sciences, Shanghai 201315, China; [f] Division of Internal Medicine, University Hospital of Basel, University of Basel, Basel, Switzerland; [g] Heart Centre Department, King Faisal Specialist Hospital & Research Center, Riyadh, Kingdom of Saudi Arabia; [h] Department of Translational Medical Sciences, "Federico II" School of Medicine, "Federico II" University of Naples, Via Pansini 5, Naples 80131, Italy; [i] Internal and Subintensive Medicine Department, Azienda Ospedaliero-Universitaria "Ospedali Riuniti", Ancona, Italy; [j] Department of Advanced Biomedical Sciences, Federico II University of Naples, Via Pansini 5, Naples I-80138, Italy; [k] Section of Respiratory Diseases, Department of Clinical Medicine and Surgery, Federico II University, Naples, Italy; [l] Centre for Rare Respiratory Diseases, Monaldi Hospital, Via Leonardo Bianchi, Naples 80131, Italy; [m] Division of Cardiology, Cardarelli Hospital, Via A. Cardarelli, 9, Naples 80131, Italy; [n] Centre for Pulmonary Hypertension, Thoraxklinik at Heidelberg University Hospital

* Corresponding author. Department of Translational Medical Sciences, "Federico II" School of Medicine, "Federico II" University of Naples, Via Pansini 5, Naples 80131, Italy.
E-mail address: alberto_marra@hotmail.it
Twitter: @alberto_marra (A.M.M.)

Heart Failure Clin 16 (2020) 317–330
https://doi.org/10.1016/j.hfc.2020.03.004
1551-7136/20/© 2020 Elsevier Inc. All rights reserved.

INTRODUCTION

Pulmonary embolism (PE), along with deep vein thrombosis (DVT), is the clinical manifestation of venous thromboembolism (VTE).[1] Acute PE is the third most common acute cardiovascular condition,[2] and its prevalence tends to grow over time.[3] PE is particularly prevalent in elderly patients,[4] leading to an estimated annual cost of 8.5 billion euros in the European Union.[5] Acute PE is burdened by remarkable mortality, up to 34% in severely ill patients presenting with hemodynamic instability.[6] However, when correctly diagnosed and promptly treated, acute PE is associated with a mortality close to 7% of patients.[7] On the other hand, the development of new imaging and biochemical tools has led to an increase in overdiagnosis of PE, which is likely to generate significant costs for health care systems.[8] Given this magnitude, special attention should be paid to ensuring that an accurate diagnosis is made within a reasonable time. Last but not least, PE might develop into chronic thromboembolic pulmonary hypertension (CTEPH), which is also burdened by remarkable morbidity and mortality.[9] Taken all together, optimal background knowledge of PE diagnosis and management and its complications should belong to all physicians, in particular, those daily dealing with acutely ill patients.

Throughout this review, 5 burning questions are addressed concerning those issues that might dramatically impact the management of PE patients, respectively:

1. Cardiac ultrasound and PE
2. Biomarkers in PE: is there something beyond D-dimer?
3. Risk stratification (RS) strategies in PE
4. Thrombolysis: to be or not to be?
5. CTEPH screening after an acute PE

CARDIAC ULTRASOUND AND PULMONARY EMBOLISM

Echocardiography is the most available, bedside, low-cost diagnostic procedure for patients with PE. Acute PE is responsible for the increase in right ventricle (RV) pressure/volume and eventually RV dysfunction. The RV is a complex structure whose evaluation poses a diagnostic challenge. For all of these reasons, there is not a single strong parameter that can be considered diagnostic itself, but there is a cluster of parameters that can lead to the suspicion of PE. The negative predictive value of echocardiography for the diagnosis of acute PE is 40% to 50%, and a negative result cannot exclude it. Transthoracic echocardiography (TTE) can visualize intracardiac thrombi (right atrium/RV) that occur in about 5% of patients and very seldom in the pulmonary arteries (Fig. 1). Transesophageal echocardiography (TEE) can detect thrombus in the central pulmonary artery (main, right, and left artery) but with a sensitivity of 30% in unselected populations.[10]

The most useful parameters for the diagnosis of PE are reported in Table 1. RV enlargement is used for the disease stratification but is present only in 25% of cases.[11] Besides, RV dilation can be also found in patients with significant left ventricular dysfunction or valvular disease. RV overload can help in the differential diagnosis between PE and RV hypokinesia/akinesia, such as in RV infarction.

A relatively new 2-dimensional RV speckle-tracking echocardiography has been clearly involved in patients with PE related to the increased afterload of the RV. According to recent studies, there is a good relationship between RV global longitudinal strain (GLS) with outcomes and response to therapy in pulmonary hypertension (PH).[12] However, there is no agreement among different investigators in the relationship between RV strain and in-hospital and long-term mortality.[13,14] The persistence of RV free-wall GLS impairment after PE correlates with worse prognosis.[15]

As general consent, because of the limited specificity of the TTE, invasiveness of TEE, and low sensitivity for both procedures, echocardiography is not considered a routine methodology to rule out PE.[16] Although echocardiography is nondiagnostic for PE, it can still provide important

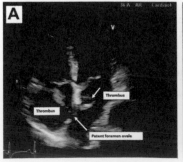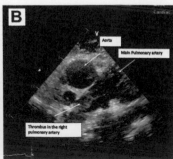

Fig. 1. TTE (*A*) and TEE (*B*) show a large horseshoe-shaped clot in the right ventricle and right atrium straddling the patent foramen ovale and arriving up to the left atrium and left ventricle.

Table 1 Echocardiographic parameters for the diagnosis of pulmonary embolism	
Window	**Parameters**
Long axis	Dilated RV
4-Chamber view	Basal diameter RV/left ventricle >1 RV basal diameter >41 mm RV middiameter >35 mm McConnell sign: akinesia of the mid free wall but normal motion at the apex (present in 10%–20% of the patients)
Parasternal short axis	Flattened interventricular septum (D-shape)
Subcostal	Dilated inferior vena cava (>21 mm) and noncollapsible during inspiration
Short axis	60/60 sign: acceleration time on pulsed wave in right ventricle outflow tract <60 ms and mid systolic notch Mild to moderate increase in pulmonary systolic pressure at the tricuspid valve (>30 and <60 mm Hg)
4-Chamber view	Reduced tricuspid annular systolic excursion by M-mode <16 mm
4-Chamber view	Decreased S′ velocity (<9.5 cm/s)
4-Chamber view	RV thrombus

information by helping to exclude other causes of severe heart dysfunction (acute left ventricular dysfunction, tamponade, acute valvular disease, and aortic dissection) and/or right-to-left shunt through a patent foramen ovale and the presence of thrombi, which are both related to increased mortality in patients with PE[17] (**Figs. 2–5**).

BIOMARKERS IN PULMONARY EMBOLISM: IS THERE SOMETHING BEYOND D-DIMER?
Biomarkers in the Right Context

Clinical symptoms and signs of PE are not specific; therefore, an unmet need of clinicians in the clinical practice is to have useful tools helping in performing fast and accurate diagnosis of PE. Following the definition of the *Biomarkers and Surrogate End Point Working Group*, a biomarker can be defined as "*a characteristic that is objectively measured and evaluated as an indicator of normal biological processes, pathogenic processes, or pharmacologic responses to a therapeutic intervention.*"[18] In addition, 3 criteria have been recently defined to consider a biomarker useful in the clinical context: (i) the biomarker has to be an accurate, repeated measurement, possible to measure with a reasonable cost and in short time; (ii) the biomarker must provide information not already available from a careful clinical assessment; and (iii) the biomarker should support the clinician in decision making.[19,20] Accordingly, biomarkers can derive from blood, urine, genetics, imaging, and biopsies. For the aim of this review, the authors focus only on circulating biomarkers. Furthermore, based on available evidence, the authors have divided into 2 categories the usefulness of clinical biomarkers in PE: (i) diagnosis; and (ii) RS.

Diagnosis of Pulmonary Embolism
D-dimer
D-dimer is a fibrin degradation product, resulted from the degradation of blood clot by plasmin (the main fibrinolysis enzyme).[21] Specifically, D-dimer is made of 2 D-fragments of the fibrin joined by a cross-link. D-dimer levels are usually not detectable in human blood plasma, and the presence of D-dimer indicates the activation of coagulation process. However, because the coagulation process can be activated by several different processes (eg, inflammation, cancer, pregnancy), D-dimer has a very low specificity. Furthermore, D-dimer levels increase with age; therefore, age-adjusted cutoff levels have been suggested.

To date, it is not arguable that D-dimer is the most important biomarker in PE. In particular, D-dimer has a very high negative predictive value, and if normal levels of D-dimer are detected, the diagnosis of PE is very unlikely. For this reason, in patients with low or intermediate clinical probability of PE (based on the combination of symptoms and clinical findings through prediction scores such as Geneve score and Wells score[22]), guidelines recommend to assess D-dimer levels[1]; if D-dimer is negative, this biomarker is enough to rule out the presence of PE. On the other hand, in the presence of a high level of D-dimer, it is necessary to perform a computed tomographic (CT) pulmonary angiogram. Using this strategy, it has been demonstrated that about

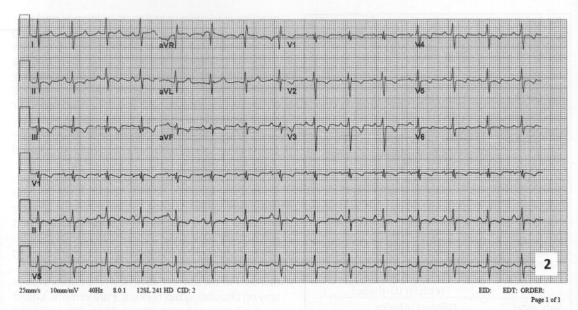

25mm/s 10mm/mV 40Hz 8.0.1 12SL 241 HD CID: 2   EID: EDT: ORDER:

Page 1 of 1

Fig. 2. A 20-year-old male patient diagnosed with intermediate-high risk, massive PE, and the presence of a mass in the RV. Upon arrival at the emergency department, the electrocardiogram showed SR. S1Q3T3 pattern of acute cor pulmonale (McGinn-White sign). Large S wave in lead I, a Q wave in lead III, and an inverted T wave in lead III together indicate acute right heart strain.

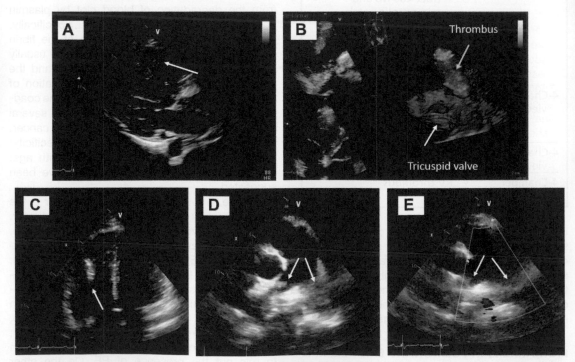

Fig. 3. Cardiac ultrasound of a 20-year-old male patient diagnosed with intermediate-high risk, massive PE, and the presence of a mass in the RV. (*A*) The RV was enlarged, and a big thrombus was seen proximal to the apex (*arrows*). (*B*) Three-dimensional echocardiogram of the RV and thrombus. (*C*) Four-chamber view showing RV enlargement with thrombus (*arrows*). (*D*) Completely obstructed right and left pulmonary artery (*arrows*). (*E*) No systolic flow in the pulmonary branches (*arrows*).

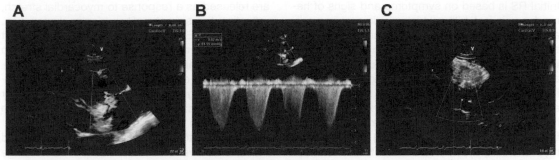

Fig. 4. Cardiac ultrasound of a 20-year-old male patient diagnosed with intermediate-high-risk PE. (*A*) Tricuspid regurgitation (TR) from the long axis for the RV. (*B*) Doppler of the TR with intense signal and triangular shape. (*C*) Dilated inferior vena cava 23 mm, noncollapsible.

30% of patients with a suspected PE in the emergency department can be safely ruled out after a negative D-dimer. D-dimer performances, however, are strongly dependent on the adopted assay. Notably, because D-dimer levels increase with age, its specificity in PE diagnosis decreases.[23] For this reason, it has been suggested to use age-adjusted cutoff levels, instead of the cutoff of 500 mg/L,[24,25] with an increase of about 25% of the number of patients ruled out without further tests.[26]

Emerging biomarkers

i. Micro-RNA (miRNA): miRNAs are circulating, noncoding RNA with a regulatory role in several processes, such as differentiation and apoptosis.[27] Because of its stability, recent research has focused on miRNAs as a novel noninvasive diagnostic biomarker of various diseases, including PE.[28,29] Recently, 2 metaanalyses have evaluated all available literature, showing that miRNAs may be considered a novel diagnostic biomarker for VTE, identifying miR-134 as the most extensive and reliable, with an average sensitivity of 0.82 and an average specificity of 0.83, with an area under the curve of 0.89.

ii. Pentraxin-3: recently, a small study involving 157 PE patients showed that pentraxin-3, an acute-phase reaction protein in inflammation derived from the pentraxin protein family (such as C-reactive protein[30]), relates to the Wells score, with higher levels in patients with high to moderate risk. Furthermore, it is associated with prognosis in PE.

iii. Lipidomic: clinical lipidomic studies lipid profiles, pathways, and networks by characterizing and quantifying the complete spectrum of lipidomes in blood samples of patients.[31] Recently, it has been demonstrated that lipidomic profiles of patients with acute lung diseases are different from healthy subjects; besides, disease-specific portions of lipidomics among patients with PE have been demonstrated, in particular when compared with patients with other pulmonary diseases (eg, acute exacerbation of obstructive pulmonary disease or severe acute pneumonia).[31] Further studies are needed to evaluate the use of this novel strategy in the clinical context.

Risk Stratification of Pulmonary Embolism

Once PE has been diagnosed, RS is due to allocate each patient to the appropriate treatment.[1]

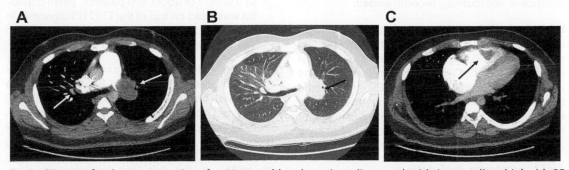

Fig. 5. CT scan of pulmonary arteries of a 20-year-old male patient diagnosed with intermediate-high risk PE shows massive bilateral PE with PH and RV strain. (*A*) Mediastinal window. (*B*) Pulmonary window (*arrows* indicate pulmonary artery thrombus). (*C*) Right ventricular thrombus (*arrow*).

Initial RS is based on symptoms and signs of hemodynamic instability, which requires an immediate emergency diagnostic and therapeutic strategy; on the other hand, patients with a situation of hemodynamic stability require further risk assessment, based on clinical, imaging, and circulating biomarkers (mostly related to RV function and myocardial injury), and presence of comorbidities. Among circulating biomarkers, 3 groups of biomarkers can be considered: (i) biomarkers of myocardial injury; (ii) biomarkers of right ventricular dysfunction; and (iii) other biomarkers.

Myocardial injury

Troponins Elevated troponins (defined as a detected value above the normal limits of the assay used) can be found in between 30% and 60% of the patients with a diagnosis of PE. An elevation in troponin levels is associated with an increased risk of mortality, identifying patients with high risk of short-term death and adverse outcome.[32] As for D-dimer as well as for troponins, the use of age-adjusted cutoff has been suggested.[33]

Based on this evidence, together with the simplified Pulmonary Embolism Severity Index (sPESI),[34] European Society of Cardiology (ESC) guidelines recommend assessing troponins levels in hemodynamically stable patients with PE, to distinguish between intermediate- to high-risk (if troponins positive) and intermediate- to low-risk (if troponins negative) patients, with a possible rescue reperfusion treatment in the first group if necessary.[1]

In regard to cutoffs, the lower detection limits for myocardial ischemia reported by the manufacturer should be adopted for troponins in the setting of PE.[35]

Myoglobin It has been demonstrated that sex-specific myoglobin levels are elevated in serum on admission in patients with PE, predicting in-hospital mortality.[36] However, its use in clinical practice is not routinely recommended.

Heart-type fatty acid-binding protein It has been demonstrated that heart-type fatty acid-binding protein (H-FABP), an early marker of myocardial injury, is associated with poor short-term outcome and mortality in patients with PE.[37–39] In some small pilot studies, H-FABP levels showed superiority to troponins, natriuretic peptides, and myoglobin in prediction of short-term outcomes.[40,41]

Right ventricular dysfunction

B-type natriuretic peptides B-type natriuretic peptide (BNP) and N-terminal proBNP (NT-proBNP) are released as a response to myocardial stretch, reflecting the severity of ventricular dysfunction. Notably, in PE, it has been demonstrated that levels of natriuretic peptides are related closer to right ventricular dysfunction than to left dysfunction.[42] High concentrations of BNP or NT-proBNP distinguish between PE patients at higher risk of complicated in-hospital course and death and those with a better prognosis.[43]

With regard to the cutoffs, it has been suggested that a BNP level of less than 50 pg/mL for triage assay was able to predict positive outcome in PE patients (lower than those used in congestive heart failure),[44] whereas for NT-proBNP, a cutoff between 500 and 600 pg/mL has been suggested.[45,46]

Other biomarkers

i. Lactate: as result of an imbalance among tissue oxygen demand and supply, elevated levels of lactate (>2 mmol/L) have been associated with poor outcome in PE patients.[47,48]
ii. Renal function: a decreased renal function estimated with glomerular filtration rate, and increased levels of creatinine are related to poor short-term outcomes as well as other biomarkers of acute kidney damage (ie, cystatin C and neutrophil gelatinase–associated lipocalin).[49,50]
iii. Hyponatremia: It has been shown that the presence of hyponatremia is associated with poor outcome in patients with acute PE.[51,52]
iv. Copeptin and adrenomedullin (ADM): Midregional proadrenomedullin (MR-pro-ADM) and copeptin, vasopressin-related biomarkers of which levels increase with stress, hypotension, and low CO, have been reported to be associated with poor outcome in PE.[53] In particular, copeptin and MR-pro-ADM were independent predictors of PE-related mortality, but they were not independent predictors of PE-related complications. In a post hoc analysis of a cohort of about 800 patients, when copeptin was used on top of the ESC RS algorithm in intermediate- to high-risk patients, copeptin was able to improve RS of PE patients.[54]

In summary, despite a large number of biomarkers that have been investigated in PE, to date, only a few of them can be considered useful in the clinical setting and able to modify the decision process in medical practice. It is not arguable that D-dimer represents the gold-standard circulating biomarker in the diagnostic process of PE, with its ability in the rule out patients with low-intermediate clinical probability of PE, or when PE is unlikely. On the other hand, troponins and brain natriuretic peptides have shown their usefulness in the RS of PE, with a pivotal role in the decision process of the treatment strategy of the patient; indeed, because of their high negative predictive value for adverse outcomes, low cardiac troponins and natriuretic peptides discriminate low-risk patients.[55]

To date, PE represents a typical condition in which a multimarker strategy, with the combination of clinical, imaging, and circulating biomarkers, appears to be the best strategy, as it has been demonstrated in several other clinical settings.[56]

RISK STRATIFICATION STRATEGIES IN PULMONARY EMBOLISM

RS of the severity and mortality owing to PE is a crucial part of everyday clinical engagement of hospitalists.[57,58] Therapeutic approaches are not unambiguous, so mastering an accurate and rapid assessment patients' PE-specific risk factors and immediate implementation of therapy are of uttermost importance in order to reduce related morbidity and lethality.[59,60]

PE mortality risks have conventionally been divided into high, intermediate (high/low), and low level. Evaluating patient's hemodynamic state (shock, severe hypotension, and similar) and right ventricular dysfunction/damage (RVD), which allow discriminating between high and not high risk, is rather unequivocal. Assessment of moderate-risk acute PE subtypes, however, are challenging and involve a variety of supporting diagnostic steps in a differentiated algorithm, which can and should be individually tailored to a given clinical situation and patient's (especially comorbidity) profile. In most cases, PE is a consequence of DVT; therefore, patients should be considered holistically.[61] Because of the acuteness and seriousness of PE, clinicians widely reach out to objective predictive scales, such as Wells, Geneva, or YEARS score.[26,62,63] However, these are to be viewed as solely supportive tools, because they do not reflect the complexity of the cases.

Further measures toward RS partially overlap with diagnostics and can be divided into laboratory testing, imaging, and clinical characteristics of the patient.[64] These 3 pillars reflect the 3 main causalities for early mortality: extent of the pulmonary circulation, associated RVD, and comorbidities.[65]

As discussed in the previous section, most valuable laboratory tests for RS include general (eg, lactate), RVD (eg, BNP), and cardiac (myocardial damage) biomarkers. Despite the fact that mostly the latter are included in the current PE risk classification, the remaining ones are of value for a comprehensive decision on further action and provide a base for recoalescence monitoring.

Although CT of the pulmonary arteries is the gold-standard diagnostic procedure, it also provides information for RS, for example, right ventricular load, (non)-movable RV clots. Similar and additional parameters can be collected via further, but inferior appliances, such as lower limb ultrasound (sensitivity 90%, specificity 95%, false positives in incomplete vein compression), ventilation and perfusion scintigraphy (insensitivity consecutively to ventilation disorders), CT angiography (positive predictive value for high and intermediate PE risk: 92%–96%; for low: 58%; negative predictive value for low and intermediate PE risk: 96% and 89%; for high: 60%), magnetic resonance angiography, echocardiography, depending on their availability and clinical condition of the patient.[66–68] Novel technologies, such as "dual-energy" imaging, "high-pitch" techniques, or monoenergetic reconstruction, are beneficial in order to further improve image quality and diagnostics.[69]

Patient-specific factors go beyond clinical symptoms and often coincide with comorbidities, especially prothrombolitic, CTEPH, hormonal (including antihormonal therapy in cancer survivors), cardiorhythmic and oncologic conditions, as well as postsurgical cases.[70,71] Pregnant patients require special consideration and approach.[72] Thus, a careful anamnesis is imperative and just as important as above-mentioned methods.

The current ESC algorithm[1] sets up 4 risk groups of PE patients: high, intermediate high, intermediate low, and low risk. This distinction can be made with 4 main diagnostic tools: hemodynamic instability combined with RV dysfunction is always to be considered high risk, independently of the PESI score or cardiac markers (troponin). If the patient is stable, there is no RV dysfunction, and the PESI score is not higher than 2, there is no obligation of measuring the troponins, and the patient is to be categorized as low risk. In the case of a PESI score III to IV, the patient is at intermediate risk. If there is an RV dysfunction or an elevated troponin level accompanying the PESI score of III to IV, intermediate-high risk is present. In case of one or both being negative, an intermediate-low risk is present. Thus, combined risk markers are the sPESI, evidence of RV dysfunction, and evidence of myocardial ischemia. If the latter two are positive, these are patients with intermediate-high risk. These patients are potential candidates for thrombolysis, either systemically or with interventional procedures (**Fig. 6**).

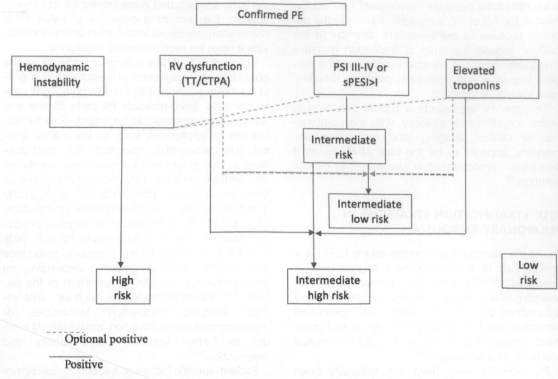

Fig. 6. RS algorithm of the severity and mortality owing to PE. TT, transthoracic echocardiography.

So far, depending on signs of RV dysfunction and/or myocardial damage, patients were differentiated as per "intermediate" and "low" mortality risk. For the first time in the new guidelines, the heterogeneous group of normotensive patients with "intermediate" risk is further stratified.

THROMBOLYSIS: TO PULMONARY EMBOLISM OR NOT TO PULMONARY EMBOLISM?
Thrombolysis in Pulmonary Embolism

The standard treatment for most patients with PE in the acute phase is anticoagulation with low-molecular-weight heparin (LMWH), unfractionated heparin (UFH), direct-acting oral anticoagulants (specifically, rivaroxaban and apixaban), or fondaparinux. Use of UFH is nowadays largely restricted to patients with hemodynamic instability or patients at high risk of hemodynamic decompensation in whom primary reperfusion treatment will be necessary.[1,73]

Pharmacologic thrombolysis (fibrinolysis)
Several studies have shown that fibrinolysis favors early lysis of the thrombus, with a reduction in pulmonary arterial pressure and an improvement in RVD faster than heparin in patients with acute PE.[74–76] In patients with high-risk PE (those who

associate hemodynamic instability), fibrinolysis appears to be associated with a reduction in mortality or recurrence of PE.[77] The recently published ESC guidelines for the diagnosis and management of acute PE have deeply defined hemodynamic instability in these patients, and it includes the following: (1) cardiac arrest; (2) obstructive shock (with systolic blood pressure <90 mm Hg or vasopressors requirement to achieve blood pressure ≥90 mm Hg and end-organ hypoperfusion); or (3) persistent hypotension (defined as systolic blood pressure <90 mm Hg or a drop of ≥40 mm Hg lasting longer than 15 minutes and not caused by arrhythmia, hypovolemia, or sepsis).[1] However, only a randomized clinical trial has been published to date that demonstrates the benefit of fibrinolysis in terms of survival in patients with high-risk PE; in that study, only 8 patients were randomized, and the trial was stopped because the 4 patients who received streptokinase survived and the 4 who received heparin died.[78] Therefore, currently, all PE treatment guidelines agree that fibrinolysis is the initial treatment of choice in patients with PE and hemodynamic instability.[1,78,79] Fibrinolytics with indication in PE are streptokinase, urokinase, and recombinant tissue plasminogen activator (eg, alteplase). Contraindications for fibrinolysis are listed in **Box 1**.

<table>
<tr><td>

Box 1
Absolute and relative contraindications for fibrinolysis

Absolute contraindications
- Hemorrhagic stroke or stroke of unknown origin (at any time)
- Ischemic stroke in the previous 6 months
- Lesions or neoplasms of the central nervous system
- Surgery/major trauma/head trauma in the previous 3 weeks
- Gastrointestinal bleeding in the last month
- Hemorrhagic diathesis

Relative contraindications
- Transient ischemic accident in the previous 6 months
- Oral anticoagulation
- Pregnancy or 1 week after delivery
- Noncompressible puncture site
- Traumatic resuscitation
- Refractory arterial hypertension (systolic blood pressure >180 mm Hg)
- Advanced liver disease
- Infective endocarditis
- Active peptic ulcer

</td></tr>
</table>

In patients with intermediate-risk PE (ie, without hypotension but with data of RVD), the main evidence available is the PEITHO trial. In PEITHO, the largest trial to date involving only patients with intermediate-risk PE (n = 1006), thrombolysis halved the number of patients who developed the primary outcome (a composite of death from any cause and hemodynamic decompensation or collapse within 7 days) from 5.6% with heparin to 2.6% with tenecteplase. However, this benefit extracted a high price, a 10-fold increase in hemorrhagic stroke (0.2% with heparin vs 2.0% with tenecteplase).[80–82] Previously, a randomized study compared heparin versus alteplase in patients with similar characteristics, finding that fibrinolysis reduced the incidence of treatment progression (catecholamines, rescue fibrinolysis, and similar), but without affecting mortality.[83] Interestingly, long-term follow-up (median 37.8 months) of patients included in the PEITHO trial (709 of 1006 initially randomized patients) showed that there was no reduction in mortalities, no reduction in persistent dyspnea or functional limitation, and no reduction in CTEPH among those patients who received thrombolysis.[82,84]

Therefore, current guidelines coincide in not advising onset fibrinolysis in patients with intermediate-risk PE.[1,78,79] However, "rescue" thrombolysis would be indicated in these patients if they developed instability or data of poor clinical evolution in the first hours despite anticoagulant treatment.[1,78]

Interventional thrombolysis
The goal of interventional thrombolysis is to remove the thrombus from the main pulmonary arteries and thus facilitate RV recovery and improve symptoms and survival. In patients with high-risk PE and contraindication for fibrinolysis (see **Table 1**) or in whom fibrinolysis has not been effective, surgical embolectomy is recommended in centers where such technique is available.[1,78] In selected patients, a perioperative mortality of 6% or less has been described, with an increase in the World Health Organization functional class and quality of life.[85–87]

As an alternative to surgery, percutaneous catheter-directed thrombolysis can be considered in centers with experience and available resources. Percutaneous thrombolysis can be performed mechanically (without drug administration) in patients at high risk of bleeding. Percutaneous thrombolysis can also be performed with administration of local fibrinolysis (catheter-directed fibrinolysis) in selected cases, primarily in patients with moderate-low risk of bleeding with contraindication for systemic fibrinolysis or those in which systemic fibrinolysis has proven ineffective. There are no clinical trials that have compared catheter-directed fibrinolysis with systemic fibrinolysis.[1] The acute-phase therapeutic strategies for patients with PE are summarized in **Table 2**.

CHRONIC THROMBOEMBOLIC PULMONARY HYPERTENSION SCREENING AFTER AN ACUTE PULMONARY EMBOLISM

As mentioned before, CTEPH is a fearsome chronic complication of acute PE whose hallmark is a persistent increase in pulmonary pressures that is closely linked to right heart failure and death.[9] The steric encumbrance caused by the presence of organized thromboembolic material may lead to an initial hemodynamic overload of those segments of the pulmonary circulation initially not affected by thromboembolic disease, which likely results in a chronic vascular remodeling.[88] CTEPH is a rare complication of acute PE, considering the data of a recently published systematic review reporting a pooled incidence of CTEPH after acute PE of

Table 2
Acute-phase therapeutic strategies for patients with pulmonary embolism

PE Type	Destination	Treatment
I. High-risk PE (cardiac arrest, obstructive shock, persistent hypotension)	Admission in intensive care unit	• Hemodynamic and respiratory support • Early fibrinolysis (streptokinase, urokinase, rTPA) • UFH (at least 24–48 h) • Once stabilized, continue treatment as in III
II. Intermediate-high risk PE (RV dysfunction by imaging AND cardiac enzymes WITHOUT hemodynamic instability)	Admission in intensive care unit or intermediate care unit (if available)	• UFH preferably if there is no contraindication for eventual thrombolysis (at least 24–48 h) • Subsequently, anticoagulation (LMWH, fondaparinux, rivaroxaban, or apixaban) • Monitoring: in case of instability, consider rescue fibrinolysis
III. Intermediate-low risk PE (RV dysfunction by imaging OR cardiac enzymes WITHOUT hemodynamic instability)	Acute ward admission	• Anticoagulation (LMWH, fondaparinux, rivaroxaban, or apixaban)
IV. Low-risk PE (no RV dysfunction and hemodynamically stable)	Consider early discharge (24–48 h) or short hospital admission	• Anticoagulation (LMWH, fondaparinux, rivaroxaban, or apixaban)

Abbreviation: rtPA, recombinant tissue plasminogen activator.

3.4% (95% confidence interval 2.1%–4.4%).[89] On the other hand, 25% of CTEPH patients do not present a previous acute PE.[90] If undiagnosed and left untreated, CTEPH is associated with a 3-year mortality of 30%.[91] For this reason, an accurate and prompt screening has a not-negligible clinical relevance. Whether PE survivors should undergo a systematic screening procedure for CTEPH was matter of debate. A post hoc analysis of the PEITHO trial reported that a long-term screening after PE lead to a CTEPH diagnosis only in 10 of 709 patients, although almost one-third of PE survivors were still symptomatic after 24 months of follow-up.[84] For this reason, the recently published European guidelines suggest to perform a routine clinical evaluation after 3 to 6 months of effective anticoagulation therapy.[1] This timeframe is necessary to ensure enough time for thrombi resolution.[92] In the case of persisting dyspnea or significant functional limitation, a Doppler TTE should be performed in order to assess the risk of PH. However, sometimes the symptoms of CTEPH can be subtle and misleading. For this reason, it is quite challenging to perform

a correct RS in patients who survived an acute PE. **Box 2** provides an overview of all the clinical conditions and risk factors that are associated with the development of a CTEPH after PE.

The results of cardiac ultrasounds may be integrated also with cardiopulmonary exercise test and/or with serum levels of natriuretic peptides.[1] Those patients with high probability of having PH should promptly undergo V/Q scan, and if mismatch perfusion defects are present, should be referred to a PH expert center for further diagnostic workup (Right heart catheterization (RHC)). It is crucial to establish a CTEPH diagnosis in a reasonable timeframe because different therapeutic options are available. The gold standard for CTEPH patients is pulmonary endoarterectomy (PEA), that when performed in a large-volume center, is likely to grant acceptable survival rates.[1] When PEA cannot be performed because of technical difficulties, or when CTEPH persists even after PEA, oral administration of Riociguat is indicated,[1] taking also into account its positive effects on RV size and function.[93,94] Balloon angioplasty should be considered alone or in addition to Riociguat.[1]

Box 2
Clinical conditions and risk factors associated with chronic thromboembolic pulmonary hypertension

Pulmonary embolism–related factors

Previous pulmonary embolism or deep venous thrombosis

Evidence of large thrombi in main pulmonary artery

Echocardiographic signs

Early signs of RV dysfunction

Ventricle-arterial shunts

Hematological conditions and/or disorders

Non-O blood group

Splenectomy

Thrombophilic disorders (antiphospholipid syndrome, high coagulation factor VIII levels)

Infections

Infected endovenous (EV) lines or pacemakers

Chronic osteomyelitis

Comorbidities

Thyroid replacement therapy

Cancers and myeloproliferative disorders

Inflammatory bowel disease

SUMMARY

Acute PE is the third most common acute cardiovascular condition, and its prevalence increases over time. With regards to diagnosis, D-dimer has a very high negative predictive value, and if normal levels of D-dimer are detected, the diagnosis of PE is very unlikely. The final diagnosis should be confirmed by CT scan. However, echocardiography is the most available, bedside, low-cost, diagnostic procedure for patients with PE. RS is of utmost importance and is mainly based on hemodynamic status of the patient. Thus, patients with PE and hemodynamic stability require further risk assessment, based on clinical symptoms, imaging, and circulating biomarkers (mainly NT-proBNP and troponin). Finally, in the case of persisting dyspnea during follow-up of a patient with PE, a TTE should be performed in order to assess the risk of PH.

DISCLOSURE

The authors have nothing to disclose.

REFERENCES

1. Konstatinides SV, Meyer G, Becattini C, et al. 2019 ESC guidelines for the diagnosis and management of acute pulmonary embolism developed in collaboration with the European Respiratory Society (ERS). Eur Heart J 2019;41(4):543–603.
2. Raskob GE, Angchaisuksiri P, Blanco AN, et al. ISTH Steering Committee for World Thrombosis Day. Thrombosis: a major contributor to global disease burden. Arterioscler Thromb Vasc Biol 2014;34: 2363–71.
3. Keller K, Hobohm L, Ebner M, et al. Trends in thrombolytic treatment and outcomes of acute pulmonary embolism in Germany. Eur Heart J 2020;41(4):522–9.
4. Wendelboe AM, Raskob GE. Global burden of thrombosis: epidemiologic aspects. Circ Res 2016; 118:1340–7.
5. Barco S, Woersching AL, Spyropoulos AC, et al. European Union-28: an annualised cost-of-illness model for venous thromboembolism. Thromb Haemost 2016;115:800–8.
6. Cohen AT, Agnelli G, Anderson FA, et al. VTE Impact Assessment Group in Europe (VITAE). Venous thromboembolism (VTE) in Europe. The number of VTE events and associated morbidity and mortality. Thromb Haemost 2007;98:756–64.
7. Bělohlávek J, Dytrych V, Linhart A. Pulmonary embolism, part I: epidemiology, risk factors and risk stratification, pathophysiology, clinical presentation, diagnosis and nonthrombotic pulmonary embolism. Exp Clin Cardiol 2013;18:129–38.
8. Wiener RS, Schwartz LM, Woloshin S. Time trends in pulmonary embolism in the United States: evidence of overdiagnosis. Arch Intern Med 2011; 171:831–7.
9. Kim NH, Delcroix M, Jais X, et al. Chronic thromboembolic pulmonary hypertension. Eur Respir J 2019; 53 [pii:1801915].
10. Cohen R, Loarte P, Navarro V, et al. Echocardiographic findings in pulmonary embolism: an important guide for the management of the patient. World Journal of Cardiovascular Diseases 2012;2: 161–4. https://doi.org/10.4236/wjcd.2012.23027.
11. Kurnicka K, Lichodziejewska B, Goliszek S, et al. Echocardiographic pattern of acute pulmonary embolism: analysis of 511 consecutive patients. J Am Soc Echocardiogr 2016;29:907–13.
12. Haeck ML, Scherptong RW, Marsan NA, et al. Prognostic value of right ventricular longitudinal peak systolic strain in patients with pulmonary hypertension. Circ Cardiovasc Imaging 2012;5:628–36.
13. Khemasuwan D, Yingchoncharoen T, Tunsupon P, et al. Right ventricular echocardiographic parameters are associated with mortality after acute pulmonary embolism. J Am Soc Echocardiogr 2015;28: 355–62.

14. Platz E, Hassanein AH, Shah A, et al. Regional right ventricular strain pattern in patients with acute pulmonary embolism. Echocardiography 2012;29:464–70.

15. Vitarelli A, Barillà F, Capotosto L, et al. Right ventricular function in acute pulmonary embolism: a combined assessment by three-dimensional and speckle-tracking echocardiography. J Am Soc Echocardiogr 2014;27:329–38.

16. Leibowitz D. Role of echocardiography in the diagnosis and treatment of acute pulmonary thromboembolism. J Am Soc Echocardiogr 2001;14:921–6.

17. Konstantinides S, Geibel A, Kasper W, et al. Patent foramen ovale is an important predictor of adverse outcome in patients with major pulmonary embolism. Circulation 1998;97:1946–51.

18. Biomarkers Definitions Working Group. Biomarkers and surrogate endpoints: preferred definitions and conceptual framework. Clin Pharmacol Ther 2001;69:89–95.

19. Morrow DA, de Lemos JA. Benchmarks for the assessment of novel cardiovascular biomarkers. Circulation 2007;115:949–52.

20. Salzano A, Marra AM, D'Assante R. Biomarkers and imaging: complementary or subtractive? Heart Fail Clin 2019;15:321–31.

21. Linkins LA, Takach Lapner S. Review of D-dimer testing: good, bad, and ugly. Int J Lab Hematol 2017;39(Suppl 1):98–103.

22. Wells PS, Anderson DR, Rodger M, et al. Excluding pulmonary embolism at the bedside without diagnostic imaging: management of patients with suspected pulmonary embolism presenting to the emergency department by using a simple clinical model and d-dimer. Ann Intern Med 2001;135:98–107.

23. Righini M, Goehring C, Bounameaux H, et al. Effects of age on the performance of common diagnostic tests for pulmonary embolism. Am J Med 2000;109:357–61.

24. Righini M, Van Es J, Den Exter PL, et al. Age-adjusted D-dimer cutoff levels to rule out pulmonary embolism: the ADJUST-PE study. JAMA 2014;311:1117–24.

25. Woller SC, Stevens SM, Adams DM, et al. Assessment of the safety and efficiency of using an age-adjusted D-dimer threshold to exclude suspected pulmonary embolism. Chest 2014;146:1444–51.

26. van der Hulle T, Cheung WY, Kooij S, et al. Simplified diagnostic management of suspected pulmonary embolism (the YEARS study): a prospective, multicentre, cohort study. Lancet 2017;390:289–97.

27. Bartel DP. MicroRNAs: genomics, biogenesis, mechanism, and function. Cell 2004;116:281–97.

28. Deng HY, Li G, Luo J, et al. MicroRNAs are novel non-invasive diagnostic biomarkers for pulmonary embolism: a meta-analysis. J Thorac Dis 2016;8:3580–7.

29. Xiang Q, Zhang HX, Wang Z, et al. The predictive value of circulating microRNAs for venous thromboembolism diagnosis: a systematic review and diagnostic meta-analysis. Thromb Res 2019;181:127–34.

30. Mantovani A, Garlanda C, Doni A, et al. Pentraxins in innate immunity: from C-reactive protein to the long pentraxin PTX3. J Clin Immunol 2008;28:1–13.

31. Gao D, Zhang L, Song D, et al. Values of integration between lipidomics and clinical phenomes in patients with acute lung infection, pulmonary embolism, or acute exacerbation of chronic pulmonary diseases: a preliminary study. J Transl Med 2019;17:162.

32. Becattini C, Vedovati MC, Agnelli G. Prognostic value of troponins in acute pulmonary embolism: a meta-analysis. Circulation 2007;116:427–33.

33. Kaeberich A, Seeber V, Jiménez D, et al. Age-adjusted high-sensitivity troponin T cut-off value for risk stratification of pulmonary embolism. Eur Respir J 2015;45:1323–31.

34. Lankeit M, Jiménez D, Kostrubiec M, et al. Predictive value of the high-sensitivity troponin T assay and the simplified Pulmonary Embolism Severity Index in hemodynamically stable patients with acute pulmonary embolism: a prospective validation study. Circulation 2011;124:2716–24.

35. Kucher N, Goldhaber SZ. Cardiac biomarkers for risk stratification of patients with acute pulmonary embolism. Circulation 2003;108:2191–4.

36. Pruszczyk P, Bochowicz A, Kostrubiec M, et al. Myoglobin stratifies short-term risk in acute major pulmonary embolism. Clin Chim Acta 2003;338(1–2):53–6.

37. Dellas C, Lobo JL, Rivas A, et al. Risk stratification of acute pulmonary embolism based on clinical parameters, H-FABP and multidetector CT. Int J Cardiol 2018;265:223–8.

38. Bajaj A, Rathor P, Sehgal V, et al. Risk stratification in acute pulmonary embolism with heart-type fatty acid-binding protein: a meta-analysis. J Crit Care 2015;30:1151.e1-7.

39. Dellas C, Puls M, Lankeit M, et al. Elevated heart-type fatty acid-binding protein levels on admission predict an adverse outcome in normotensive patients with acute pulmonary embolism. J Am Coll Cardiol 2010;55:2150–7.

40. Kaczyñska A, Pelsers MM, Bochowicz A, et al. Plasma heart-type fatty acid binding protein is superior to troponin and myoglobin for rapid risk stratification in acute pulmonary embolism. Clin Chim Acta 2006;371(1–2):117–23.

41. Bajaj A, Rathor P, Sehgal V, et al. Prognostic value of biomarkers in acute non-massive pulmonary embolism: a systematic review and meta-analysis. Lung 2015;193:639–51.

42. Pasha SM, Klok FA, van der Bijl N, et al. NT-pro-BNP levels in patients with acute pulmonary embolism are correlated to right but not left ventricular volume and function. Thromb Haemost 2012;108:367–72.

43. Klok FA, Mos IC, Huisman MV. Brain-type natriuretic peptide levels in the prediction of adverse outcome in patients with pulmonary embolism: a systematic review and meta-analysis. Am J Respir Crit Care Med 2008;178:425–30.

44. Jovanovic L, Subota V, Stavric M, et al. Biomarkers for the prediction of early pulmonary embolism related mortality in spontaneous and provoked thrombotic disease. Clin Chim Acta 2019;492: 78–83.

45. Agterof MJ, Schutgens RE, Snijder RJ, et al. Out of hospital treatment of acute pulmonary embolism in patients with a low NT-proBNP level. J Thromb Haemost 2010;8:1235–41.

46. Lankeit M, Jiménez D, Kostrubiec M, et al. Validation of N-terminal pro-brain natriuretic peptide cut-off values for risk stratification of pulmonary embolism. Eur Respir J 2014;43:1669–77.

47. Vanni S, Viviani G, Baioni M, et al. Prognostic value of plasma lactate levels among patients with acute pulmonary embolism: the thrombo-embolism lactate outcome study. Ann Emerg Med 2013;61: 330–8.

48. Vanni S, Nazerian P, Bova C, et al. Comparison of clinical scores for identification of patients with pulmonary embolism at intermediate-high risk of adverse clinical outcome: the prognostic role of plasma lactate. Intern Emerg Med 2017;12:657–65.

49. Kostrubiec M, Pływaczewska M, Jiménez D, et al. The prognostic value of renal function in acute pulmonary embolism–a multi-centre cohort study. Thromb Haemost 2019;119:140–8.

50. Kostrubiec M, Łabyk A, Pedowska-Włoszek J, et al. Neutrophil gelatinase-associated lipocalin, cystatin C and eGFR indicate acute kidney injury and predict prognosis of patients with acute pulmonary embolism. Heart 2012;98:1221–8.

51. Zhou XY, Chen HL, Ni SS. Hyponatremia and short-term prognosis of patients with acute pulmonary embolism: a meta-analysis. Int J Cardiol 2017;227: 251–6.

52. Scherz N1, Labarère J, Méan M, et al. Prognostic importance of hyponatremia in patients with acute pulmonary embolism. Am J Respir Crit Care Med 2010;182:1178–83.

53. Vuilleumier N, Simona A, Méan M, et al. Comparison of cardiac and non-cardiac biomarkers for risk stratification in elderly patients with non-massive pulmonary embolism. PLoS One 2016;11:e0155973.

54. Hellenkamp K, Pruszczyk P, Jiménez D, et al. Prognostic impact of copeptin in pulmonary embolism: a multicentre validation study. Eur Respir J 2018;51 [pii:1702037].

55. Pradhan NM, Mullin C, Poor HD. Biomarkers and right ventricular dysfunction. Crit Care Clin 2020; 36:141–53.

56. Salzano A, Israr MZ, Yazaki Y, et al. Combined use of trimethylamine N-oxide with BNP for risk stratification in heart failure with preserved ejection fraction: findings from the DIAMONDHFpEF study. Eur J Prev Cardiol 2019. https://doi.org/10.4236/wjcd. 2012.23027. 2047487319870355.

57. Butler SP, Quinn RJ. The clinical course of pulmonary embolism. N Engl J Med 1992;327:957–8.

58. Goldhaber SZ, Elliott CG. Acute pulmonary embolism: part II: risk stratification, treatment, and prevention. Circulation 2003;108:2834–8.

59. Becattini C, Agnelli G. Acute pulmonary embolism: risk stratification in the emergency department. Intern Emerg Med 2007;2:119–29.

60. Chatterjee S, Chakraborty A, Weinberg I, et al. Thrombolysis for pulmonary embolism and risk of all-cause mortality, major bleeding, and intracranial hemorrhage: a meta-analysis. JAMA 2014;311: 2414–21.

61. Di Nisio M, van Es N, Büller HR. Deep vein thrombosis and pulmonary embolism. Lancet 2016;388: 3060–73.

62. Penaloza A, Verschuren F, Meyer G. Comparison of the unstructured clinician gestalt, the wells score, and the revised Geneva score to estimate pretest probability for suspected pulmonary embolism. Ann Emerg Med 2013;62:117–24.e2.

63. Hendriksen JM, Geersing GJ, Lucassen WA, et al. Diagnostic prediction models for suspected pulmonary embolism: systematic review and independent external validation in primary care. BMJ 2015;351: h4438.

64. Giannitsis E, Katus HA. Risk stratification in pulmonary embolism based on biomarkers and echocardiography. Circulation 2005;112:1520–1.

65. Fesmire FM, Brown MD, Espinosa JA, et al. Critical issues in the evaluation and management of adult patients presenting to the emergency department with suspected pulmonary embolism. Ann Emerg Med 2011;57:628–52.e75.

66. Oudkerk M, van Beek EJ, Wielopolski P, et al. Comparison of contrast-enhanced magnetic resonance angiography and conventional pulmonary angiography for the diagnosis of pulmonary embolism: a prospective study. Lancet 2002;359: 1643–7.

67. Wittram C, Maher MM, Yoo AJ, et al. CT angiography of pulmonary embolism: diagnostic criteria and causes of misdiagnosis. Radiographics 2004;24: 1219–38.

68. Stein PD, Woodard PK, Weg JG, et al. Diagnostic pathways in acute pulmonary embolism: recommendations of the PIOPED II investigators. Am J Med 2006;119:1048–55.

69. Moore AJE, Wachsmann J, Chamarthy MR, et al. Imaging of acute pulmonary embolism: an update. Cardiovasc Diagn Ther 2018;8:225–43.

70. Sørensen HT, Mellemkjaer L, Steffensen FH, et al. The risk of a diagnosis of cancer after primary deep venous thrombosis or pulmonary embolism. N Engl J Med 1998;338:1169–73.

71. Rali PM, Criner GJ. Submassive pulmonary embolism. Am J Respir Crit Care Med 2018;198:588–98.

72. van der Pol LM, Tromeur C, Bistervels IM, et al. Pregnancy-adapted YEARS algorithm for diagnosis of suspected pulmonary embolism. N Engl J Med 2019;380:1139–49.

73. Peñaloza-Martínez E, Demelo-Rodríguez P, Proietti M, et al. Update on extended treatment for venous thromboembolism. Ann Med 2018;50: 666–74.

74. Miller GA, Sutton GC, Kerr IH, et al. Comparison of streptokinase and heparin in treatment of isolated acute massive pulmonary embolism. Br Med J 1971;2:681–4.

75. Goldhaber SZ, Haire WD, Feldstein ML, et al. Alteplase versus heparin in acute pulmonary embolism: randomised trial assessing right-ventricular function and pulmonary perfusion. Lancet 1993;341:507–11.

76. Becattini C, Agnelli G, Salvi A, et al. Bolus tenecteplase for right ventricle dysfunction in hemodynamically stable patients with pulmonary embolism. Thromb Res 2010;125:e82–6.

77. Wan S, Quinlan DJ, Agnelli G, et al. Thrombolysis compared with heparin for the initial treatment of pulmonary embolism: a meta-analysis of the randomized controlled trials. Circulation 2004;110: 744–9.

78. Konstantinides SV, Barco S, Lankeit M, et al. Management of pulmonary embolism: an update. J Am Coll Cardiol 2016;67:976–90.

79. Kearon C, Akl EA, Ornelas J, et al. Antithrombotic therapy for VTE disease: CHEST guideline and expert panel report. Chest 2016;149:315–52.

80. Meyer G, Vicaut E, Danays T, et al. Fibrinolysis for patients with intermediate-risk pulmonary embolism. N Engl J Med 2014;370:1402–11.

81. Eberle H, Lyn R, Knight T, et al. Clinical update on thrombolytic use in pulmonary embolism: a focus on intermediate-risk patients. Am J Health Syst Pharm 2018;75:1275–85.

82. Goldhaber SZ. PEITHO long-term outcomes study: data disrupt dogma. J Am Coll Cardiol 2017;69: 1545–8.

83. Konstantinides S, Geibel A, Heusel G, et al. Heparin plus alteplase compared with heparin alone in patients with submassive pulmonary embolism. N Engl J Med 2002;347:1143–50.

84. Konstantinides SV, Vicaut E, Danays T, et al. Impact of thrombolytic therapy on the long-term outcome of intermediate-risk pulmonary embolism. J Am Coll Cardiol 2017;69:1536–44.

85. Takahashi H, Okada K, Matsumori M, et al. Aggressive surgical treatment of acute pulmonary embolism with circulatory collapse. Ann Thorac Surg 2012;94:785–91.

86. Leacche M, Unic D, Goldhaber SZ, et al. Modern surgical treatment of massive pulmonary embolism: results in 47 consecutive patients after rapid diagnosis and aggressive surgical approach. J Thorac Cardiovasc Surg 2005;129:1018–23.

87. Aymard T, Kadner A, Widmer A, et al. Massive pulmonary embolism: surgical embolectomy versus thrombolytic therapy–should surgical indications be revisited? Eur J Cardiothorac Surg 2013;43:90–4.

88. Dorfmüller P, Günther S, Ghigna MR, et al. Microvascular disease in chronic thromboembolic pulmonary hypertension: a role for pulmonary veins and systemic vasculature. Eur Respir J 2014;44:1275–88.

89. Simonneau G, Torbicki A, Dorfmüller P, et al. The pathophysiology of chronic thromboembolic pulmonary hypertension. Eur Respir Rev 2017;26 [pii: 160112].

90. Pepke-Zaba J, Delcroix M, Lang I, et al. Chronic thromboembolic pulmonary hypertension (CTEPH): results from an international prospective registry. Circulation 2011;124:1973–81.

91. Delcroix M, Lang I, Pepke-Zaba J, et al. Long-term outcome of patients with chronic thromboembolic pulmonary hypertension: results from an international prospective registry. Circulation 2016;133: 859–71.

92. Wartski M, Collignon MA. Incomplete recovery of lung perfusion after 3 months in patients with acute pulmonary embolism treated with antithrombotic agents. THESEE Study Group. Tinzaparin ou heparin standard: evaluation dans l'Embolie Pulmonaire Study. J Nucl Med 2000;41:1043–8.

93. Marra AM, Egenlauf B, Ehlken N, et al. Change of right heart size and function by long-term therapy with riociguat in patients with pulmonary arterial hypertension and chronic thromboembolic pulmonary hypertension. Int J Cardiol 2015;195:19–26.

94. Marra AM, Halank M, Benjamin N, et al. Right ventricular size and function under riociguat in pulmonary arterial hypertension and chronic thromboembolic pulmonary hypertension (the RIVER study). Respir Res 2018;19(1):258.

Imaging Cardiovascular Emergencies
Real World Clinical Cases

Ciro Mauro, MD[a,1], Olga Vriz, MD[b,1], Luigia Romano, MD[c],
Rodolfo Citro, MD, PhD[d], Valentina Russo, MD[e], Brigida Ranieri, PhD[f],
Bandar Alamro, MD[b], Mohammed Aladmawi, MD[b], Riccardo Granata, MD[e],
Domenico Galzerano, MD, FESC[b], Michele Bellino, MD[d],
Rosangela Cocchia, MD[g], Rahul M. Mehta, MD[h],
Santo Delle Grottaglie, MD[i], Hani Alsergani, MD[b], Rajendra H. Mehta, MD[j,2],
Eduardo Bossone, MD, PhD, FCCP, FESC, FACC[g,*,2]

KEYWORDS

- Cardiovascular emergencies • Biomarkers • Transthoracic echocardiography
- Computed tomography • Magnetic resonance imaging

KEY POINTS

- Cardiovascular disease is the most prevalent and leading cause of death worldwide (17.6 million deaths/y).
- Cardiovascular emergencies represent life-threatening conditions requiring a high index of clinical suspicion.
- In an emergency scenario, a simple stepwise biomarker/imaging diagnostic algorithm may help making a prompt diagnosis and timely treatment along with related improved outcomes.

INTRODUCTION

Cardiovascular disease is the most prevalent and leading cause of death worldwide (17.6 million deaths/y).[1] In this regard, cardiovascular emergencies (CVEs) represent life-threatening conditions requiring a high index of clinical suspicion, prompt diagnosis, and timely appropriate therapeutic interventions.[2] This article discusses the biomarker/imaging diagnostic pathways of the most common CVEs through a series of real-world cases.

[a] Cardiology Division, A Cardarelli Hospital, Via Cardarelli 9, Naples I-80131, Italy; [b] Cardiology Department, Heart Centre, King Faisal Specialist Hospital & Research Centre, MBC-16, PO Box 3354, Riyadh 11211, Saudi Arabia; [c] Department of General and Emergency Radiology, A Cardarelli Hospital, Via Cardarelli 9, Naples I-80131, Italy; [d] Cardiology Unit, Cardiovascular and Thoracic Department, University Hospital "San Giovanni di Dio e Ruggi d'Aragona", Largo Città d'Ippocrate, Salerno 84131, Italy; [e] Department of Advanced Biomedical Sciences, Federico II University of Naples, Via Pansini 5, Naples I-80131, Italy; [f] IRCCS SDN, Via Gianturco 113, Naples I-80142, Italy; [g] Division of Cardiac Rehabilitation - Echo Lab, A Cardarelli Hospital, Naples, Italy; [h] ProMedica Monroe Regional Hospital, 718 North Macomb Street, Monroe, MI 48162, USA; [i] Villa dei Fiori, Corso Italia 110, Mugnano di Napoli, Naples 80018, Italy; [j] Duke Clinical Research Institute, Durham, 300 West Morgan Street, Durham, NC 27701, USA
[1] Equally contributed.
[2] Equally contributed.
* Corresponding author. Division of Cardiac Rehabilitation - Echo Lab, A Cardarelli Hospital, Via Cardarelli 9, Naples I-80131, Italy
E-mail address: eduardo.bossone@aocardarelli.it

Heart Failure Clin 16 (2020) 331–346
https://doi.org/10.1016/j.hfc.2020.03.003

BIOMARKER-IMAGING ALGORITHM STRATEGY FOR CARDIOVASCULAR EMERGENCIES

Diagnosis in CVEs often can be challenging due to a lack of typical symptoms and signs. In a majority of cases, patients may present with chest pain and/or dyspnea. In an emergency scenario, a stepwise diagnostic algorithm strategy that utilizes biomarker imaging includes comprehensive clinical evaluation (medical history/physical examination and related pretest probabilities; and a Bayesian approach), laboratory tests (mainly cardiac troponins, B-type natriuretic peptide [BNP] and N-terminal proBNP [NT-proBNP], and D-dimer),[3] and imaging methods (electrocardiogram [ECG], chest radiograph [CXR], transthoracic echocardiography [TTE], and computed tomography [CT]) (**Fig. 1**). A fast TTE (including a glimpse of the aortic arch and abdominal aorta) is strongly recommended in emergency settings. It has been demonstrated to be an accurate tool to assess cardiac structure and function along with noninvasive Doppler-derived hemodynamics.[2] Transesophageal echocardiography (TEE), if available and when there are no contraindications to it, remains a valid added imaging tool in cardiac valve and aorta diseases, intracardiac thrombus, and shunts. The key role of CT angiography, which usually is widely available and easily accessible in emergency settings, cannot be overemphasized. Among patients presenting with chest pain ECG gating, CT angiography triple rule-out strategy has been proposed in order to simultaneously assess coronary arteries (myocardial ischemia),

thoracic aorta (acute aortic syndromes/aneurysms), and pulmonary arteries (pulmonary embolism [PE]). Furthermore, CT angiography is considered first-line diagnostic imaging technique (accuracy close to 100%) in cases of clinical suspicion of traumatic aortic injury as consequence of major blunt thoracic trauma (eg high-speed motor vehicle or falling from a great height).[4] CT is not a bedside imaging modality and, compared with echocardiography, the only major limitation is the need to transfer a potentially critical patient to in a separate area of the emergency department (ED), while monitoring and supporting vital functions. Although the use of magnetic resonance imaging (MRI) in an emergency scenario remains limited (no widespread availability, time consuming, and not suitable for unstable patients), it is gaining a pivotal diagnostic role in the subacute phase in some clinical scenarios. Specifically, distinct differential features of potential prognostic relevance have been demonstrated with cardiac MRI among patients with myocarditis, takotsubo syndrome (TTS), and acute coronary syndromes,[5] and this imaging test recently has been introduced in the diagnostic algorithm recommended for patients with myocardial infarction with nonobstructive coronary arteries.[6] In addition, cardiac MRI has the highest sensitivity in detecting ventricular thrombi in subjects with reduced ventricular function or other predisposing conditions.[7] Nuclear cardiology rarely finds a definite role in management of patients with a CVE, with the only potential exception ventilation/perfusion lung scintigraphy applied in stable patients with

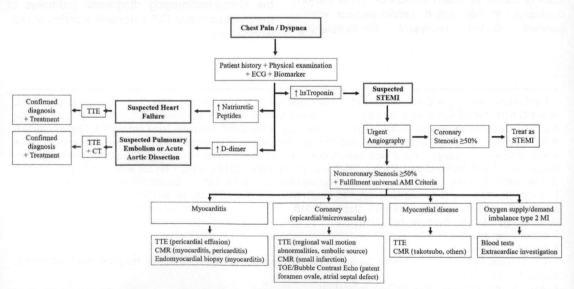

Fig. 1. Diagnostic algorithm. hs, high-sensitivity; MI, myocardial infarction; TOE, transesophageal echocardiography. (*Data from* Refs.[3,6,8,25])

suspected acute PE and contraindication to CT (eg contrast allergy or renal impairment).[8]

SPECIFIC CARDIOVASCULAR EMERGENCIES
Acute Myocardial Infarction

Despite the substantial advances in diagnostic and treatment strategies over the past decades, ischemic heart disease represents the most common cause of mortality in developed countries, accounting for approximately 1.8 million annual deaths in Europe. The current definition of myocardial infarction[9] requires the presence of acute myocardial injury defined as an elevation of cardiac troponin values with at least 1 value above the 99th percentile upper reference limit (**Box 1**). On the basis of an underling mechanism, leading to an imbalance between oxygen supply and myocardial demand, and of clinical context, myocardial infarction is classified as type I in cases of spontaneous atherosclerotic plaque rupture, ulceration, fissuring, erosion, and dissection resulting in intraluminal thrombus formation in 1 or more of the coronary arteries. Type II myocardial infarction is defined as secondary to ischemic imbalance, due, for example, to severe anemia, coronary endothelial dysfunction, coronary artery spasm, embolism, tachyarrhythmias/bradyarrhythmias, respiratory failure, hypotension, or hypertension with or without left ventricular hypertrophy. Cardiac death due to myocardial infarction is classified as type III, whereas an event associated with revascularization procedures is type IV after percutaneous coronary interventions

---

Box 1
Myocardial infarction diagnostic criteria

Detection of rise and/or fall of cardiac troponin values with at least 1 value above the 99th percentile upper reference limit and with at least 1 of the following:

- Symptoms of acute myocardial ischemia

- New ischemic ECG changes

- Development of pathologic Q waves

- Imaging evidence of new loss of viable myocardium or new regional wall motion abnormality in a pattern consistent with an ischemic etiology

- Identification of a coronary thrombus by angiography including intracoronary imaging or by autopsy

Modified from Thygesen K, Alpert JS, Jaffe AS, et al. Fourth Universal Definition of Myocardial Infarction (2018). Circulation. 2018 Nov 13;138(20):e618-e651.

---

and is type V after coronary artery bypass grafting. From a clinical point of view, myocardial infarction requires a prompt distinction based on ECG findings in ST segment elevation forms (STEMI), often suggestive of ongoing coronary artery acute occlusion, candidate to immediate reperfusion strategy, preferably through percutaneous coronary intervention. In opposite, the non ST segment elevation myocardial infarction (NSTEMI) requires a therapeutic approach that must be tailored based on risk stratification (an early invasive approach as a preferable strategy for treatment of intermediate to high-risk subsets).[6,10] Fractional flow reserve during angiography may help determine the functional significance of borderline coronary lesions that would benefit from percutaneous coronary intervention.

The role of echocardiography

In an emergency scenario, color Doppler echocardiography (transthoracic color Doppler echocardiography and TEE) when clinically indicated allows (1) identifying regional wall motion abnormalities, confirming an acute myocardial infarction (AMI) diagnosis (especially in patients presenting with atypical symptoms or confounding ECG findings); (2) quantifying systolic global function; (3) detecting and planning relative surgical treatment; and (4) identifying mechanical complications.[11] In particular, although with the widespread use of primary percutaneous coronary intervention, the overall incidence of AMI mechanical complications is now reduced between 1% and 2%, AMI mechanical complications have a dramatic outcome if not treated promptly and echocardiography is the key methodology for diagnosis. Papillary muscle rupture is associated with very high in-hospital mortality—80% in centers without on-site surgery versus 19% to 53% in centers with on-site surgery. Similarly, high in-hospital mortality is encountered in cases of free wall (20%–75%) and left ventricular septal rupture (20%–40%).[12–14]

The role of computed tomography

CT (triple rule-out strategy) may be implemented for the evaluation of patients with low risk to intermediate risk of acute coronary syndrome (acute chest pain of doubtful etiology, borderline levels of cardiac enzymes, and/or nonpathognomonic ECG changes). It has been demonstrated to convey a high sensitivity (86%–100%) along with a high negative predictive value (93%–100%).[4]

Clinical case: coronary stent thrombosis-restenosis

A 57-year-old man, a current smoker with hypertension and coronary artery disease, presented with severe chest pain and ST elevation in anterior and lateral leads on ECG at the ED (**Fig. 2**A). The patient 2 days before had arbitrarily interrupted dual-antiplatelet therapy (ticagrelor and aspirin) given for severe restenosis in the proximal segment of left anterior descending artery (treated with stent-in-stent implantation) of a stent implanted 3 years before for acute coronary syndrome. The coronary angiogram showed acute in-stent occlusion of the left anterior descending artery (**Fig. 2**B, C) and it was treated with multiple dilation with paclitaxel-coated balloon (**Fig. 2**D).

Takotsubo Syndrome

TTS is an acute clinical condition mimicking acute coronary syndrome characterized by diffuse myocardial stunning generally reversible within a few days or weeks.[15,16] Etiology is still unknown; however, high serum catecholamines spillover secondary to trigger events seem to have a key role in pathogenesis of this peculiar syndrome.[17] Owing to

its transient nature, it is thought to have a favorable prognosis, but several registries have documented a considerable number of life-threatening complications during the acute phase.[18] Echocardiography is the first-line diagnostic imaging method; it is fundamental for diagnosis, for identifying possible unfavorable mechanical complications requiring specific therapeutic management, and monitoring recovery of myocardial function.[17–19] Coronary angiography often confirms absence of significant coronary stenosis.

Clinical case: takotsubo syndrome

A 58-year-old postmenopausal woman with mood disorder and without risk factors for coronary artery disease was admitted to the ED for retrosternal chest pain occurred after the scare for risking a road crash. Anterior ST elevation at ECG (**Fig. 3**A) and akinesia of the left ventricular apical segments at bedside emergency echocardiography were detected. Patient was treated with enoxaparin,

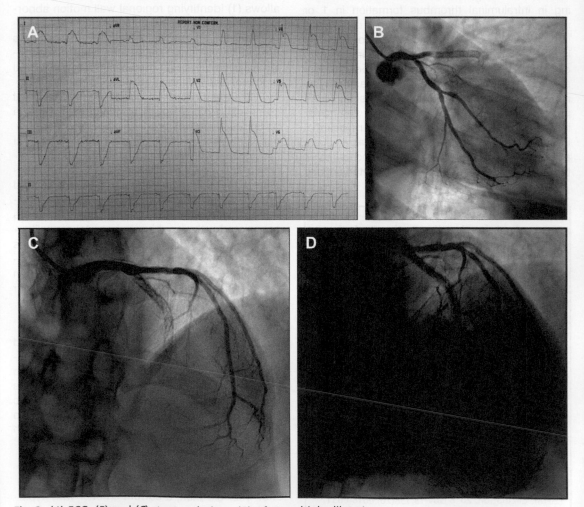

Fig. 2. (*A*) ECG. (*B*) and (*C*) stent occlusions. (*D*) After multiple dilatation.

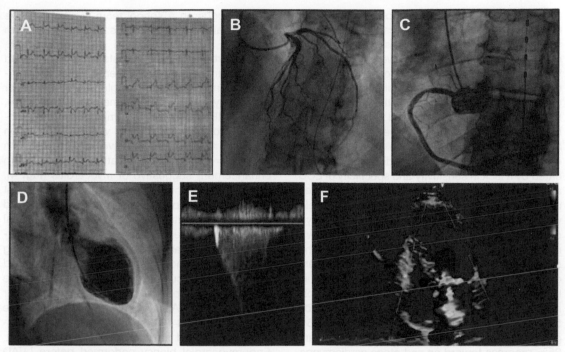

Fig. 3. (*A*) ECG with anterior ST elevation. (*B*) Left coronary artery at angiography. (*C*) Right coronary artery at angiography. (*D*) Ventriculography showing apical ballooning. (*E*) Continuous-wave Doppler at TTE showing intraventricular gradient. (*F*) Severe mitral functional regurgitation at TTE.

aspirin, ticagrelor, and atorvastatin and transferred to a catheter laboratory. Coronary angiography revealed normal coronary arteries (**Fig. 3**B, C) and ventriculography showed apical ballooning (**Fig. 3**D). The suspected TTS was reinforced by calculating an InterTAK Diagnostic Score of 78 points.[17] At coronary care unit admission, the patient developed dyspnea and profuse sweating. Thoracic auscultation revealed midbasal pulmonary rales and pansystolic murmur at the apex. Arterial blood pressure (BP) was 88/56 mm Hg with a Po_2 66 mm Hg and a BNP 867 pg/mL. TTE showed an ejection fraction of 40% and an intraventricular gradient of 60.52 mm Hg (**Fig. 3**E), indicative of left ventricular outflow tract obstruction (LVOTO) and systolic anterior movement of the anterior mitral leaflet with severe functional mitral regurgitation (**Fig. 3**F). Owing to the onset of the signs of hemodynamic instability, pulmonary congestion cardiogenic shock, and pulmonary edema in the patient, TTS complicated by LVOTO and mitral regurgitation was diagnosed. The patient was treated with repetitive boluses of a short-acting β-blocker, esmolol intravenous infusion, to avoid prolonged hypotensive effect, increase left ventricular filling time, and reduce intraventricular dynamic obstruction and consequently the amount of mitral regurgitation volume. Also, loop diuretics were administered with

caution. After a few hours, the symptoms reduced with improvement of hemodynamic parameters, and esmolol and diuretics were progressively withdrawn. Subsequently patient clinical conditions improved with disappearance of LVOTO and reduction of mitral regurgitation grade at echo scanning. On the fourth day, the patient was transferred in standard room of cardiology unit where she remained asymptomatic. After echocardiographic detection of significant recovery of left ventricular myocardial function (ejection fraction = 55%), the patient was discharged on the seventh day on therapy with metoprolol, ramipril, and aspirin.

Myocarditis

Myocarditis (defined as an inflammatory disease of the myocardium) represents one of the most frequent cause of dilated cardiomyopathy and sudden cardiac death.[20,21] It typically is triggered by a cardiotropic viral infection, leading to an active inflammation of myocardium. Although advances in polymerase chain reaction technology have enabled detection of enteroviruses, adenoviruses, parvovirus B19, and human herpesvirus 6 as the most common causes of acute myocarditis, several other etiologies also have been described, including HIV, Chagas disease, toxins, medications, and autoimmune phenomena. Diagnosis may be challenging. Myocarditis usually presents with heterogeneous signs and symptoms, ranging from subclinical paucisymptomatic evolution to chest pain mimicking myocardial infarction, refractory cardiogenic shock, or sudden cardiac death from ventricular fibrillation. Serum biomarkers, namely troponin I and troponin T white blood cell counts, erythrocyte sedimentation rate, and C-reactive protein (CRP) levels, may be elevated. A diagnosis of myocarditis also is complicated by a lack in sensitivity and specificity of ECG, alterations such as nonspecific ST segment changes, T-wave inversions, and ST segment elevations often comparable to acute coronary syndromes. In this contest, TTE is able to detect wall motion abnormalities (usually not correlated with a defined coronary territory) and quantify the grade of left ventricular systolic dysfunction. The natural history of myocarditis generally is unpredictable: in the presence of left ventricular dysfunction, 50% of patients have complete resolution, 25% go on to have chronic systolic dysfunction, and 25% progress toward an end-stage cardiomyopathy resulting in heart transplantation or death. Although coronary angiogram remains the gold standard to exclude obstructive coronary disease, cardiovascular MRI (CMR) is the imaging method used most frequently able to detect inflammation, edema, necrosis, and/or fibrosis within myocardial tissue.

Regarding therapies, besides supportive treatments for heart failure and arrhythmia, no specific recommendations exist but individual modulation of the immune system is a promising therapeutic strategy, as suggested by several randomized trials.[20,21]

Clinical case: acute myocarditis

A 14-year-old boy, with a 10-day history of recurrent fever (zenith 38.6°C) and evidence of pharyngitis, presented at the ED with mild exertional dyspnea and initial signs of heart failure. He had no previous background of heart disease and played soccer in a school team regularly. At the initial evaluation, vital signs were stable with adequate systolic BP, mild sinus tachycardia, and no orthopnea. Blood tests revealed elevated troponin and leukocyte number, whereas his echocardiogram showed severe global left ventricular systolic dysfunction. The same day of admission, cardiac MRI showed severe impairment of ventricular systolic function (left ventricular ejection fraction = 18%; right ventricular ejection fraction = 24%), with a pattern of gadolinium enhancement suggestive of myocarditis (**Fig. 4**). Considering the provisional diagnosis of fulminant myocarditis, the patient was promptly transferred to a tertiary hospital for further management. Initial treatment included furosemide, eplerenone, carvedilol, ramipril, and digoxin. During the following days, the hemodynamic status deteriorated despite intravenous high-dose inotropes, and the patient was implanted with a left ventricular assist device (LVAD) without complications. While still in hospital at 12 weeks after LVAD implantation, he received an orthotopic heart transplant. Endomyocardial biopsy performed before LVAD implantation and examination of the explanted heart confirmed the diagnosis of a lymphocytic myocarditis. Approximately 1 month later, the patient was safely discharged and a tight schedule of follow-up appointments was planned. After a 1-year follow-up period free of clinical events, the patient presented with fatigue and weight gain secondary to a reduced diuresis. Initial cardiac evaluation documented the occurrence of some episodes of nonsustained ventricular tachycardia. A repeated cardiac MRI study revealed moderate septal hypertrophy (end-diastolic wall thickness = 14 mm), with signs of altered tissue composition, best seen at the level of the right side of the interventricular septum, suggestive of possible cardiac transplant rejection (**Fig. 5**). Endomyocardial biopsy confirmed moderate allograft cellular rejection, which was treated successfully with standard steroids and

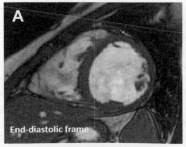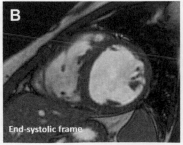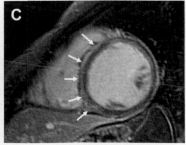

Fig. 4. Cardiac MRIs obtained in a short-axis midventricular plane and showing (*A*) and (*B*) severe biventricular dilation and systolic dysfunction by cine imaging and (*C*) areas of contrast enhancement with nonischemic pattern by late postcontrast imaging, best seen at the level of the interventricular septum (*arrows*).

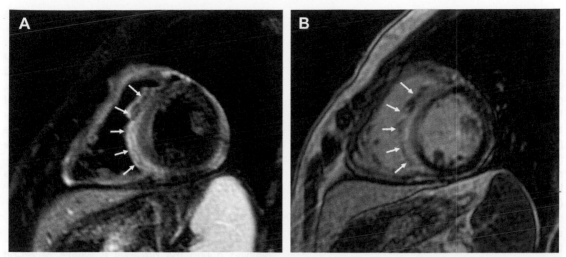

Fig. 5. Cardiac MRIs obtained in a short-axis midventricular plane and showing (*A*) areas of increased tissue signal by T2-weighted imaging (as a sign of myocardial edema) and of contrast enhancement (*B*) by late postcontrast imaging (as a sign of myocardial edema/fibrosis), best seen at the level of the right side of the interventricular septum (*arrows*).

immunosuppressive therapy protocols. At a further 5-year follow-up, the patient was stable with preserved functional capacity.

Acute Pulmonary Embolism

Acute PE—incidence from 53 per 100,00 to 162 per 100,00 population; among unselected cohort of patients, mortality rate 11.4% at 2 weeks and 17.4% at 3 months—is defined as the acute obstruction of 1 or more branches of the pulmonary artery by embolic material of extrapulmonary origin and represents the most frequent cause of cor pulmonale, with a high incidence of mortality (**Table 1**). In most cases, embolic material comes from deep venous thrombosis (DVT); for this reason, according to European Society of Cardiology guidelines, PE and DVT often are included as a single pathologic and clinical entity, defined as venous thromboembolism, the third most common cardiovascular disease, with an annual incidence of 1.2 per 1000 to 2.7 per 1000.[8]

In cases of suspected acute PE, the diagnostic algorithm is based on clinical evaluation (with or without hemodynamic instability), biomarkers (D-dimer) and imaging (TTE and CT pulmonary angiography [CTPA]) (see **Fig. 1**). CTPA is the method of choice for imaging the pulmonary vasculature in patients with suspected PE (sensitivity of 83% and specificity 96%). In addition, TEE may be useful in order to detect emboli in right heart and proximal pulmonary arteries; while bilateral venous compression ultrasonography may be useful in order to detect DVT.[22–24]

Clinical case: massive pulmonary embolism
A 62-year-old woman presented to the ED complaining of shortness of breath on minimal exertion and cough. Recent spinal cord surgery was registered on medical history. She was tachycardic, with BP, 110/65 mm Hg, and was hypoxic on room air (saturation: Po_2 87%). Laboratory results were white blood cell count, 10.97x 10^9/L; hemoglobin (Hb), 11.7 g/L; D-dimer, 2.55 μg/mL fibrinogen-equivalent units (normal value 0.5); proBNP, 1.545 pg/mL; and creatinine, 69 mmol/L. ECG showed sinus tachycardia (heart rate [HR] 120 BPM) and S1Q3T3 pattern, suggesting PE; CXR was

Table 1
Mortality rate of acute pulmonary embolism

Massive Pulmonary Embolism	Mortality (%)
Overall	18 to 65
Treated	20
With cardiogenic shock	25 to 30
With resuscitation	65
Submassive PE	5 to 25
PE with mobile thrombi in right heart chambers	Up to 27
Small PE	Up to 1

Data from Konstantinides SV, Meyer G, Becattini C, et al.; ESC Scientific Document Group. 2019 ESC Guidelines for the diagnosis and management of acute pulmonary embolism developed in collaboration with the European Respiratory Society (ERS). Eur Heart J. 2020;41(4):543–603.

unremarkable (**Fig. 6**). TTE showed dilated right ventricle, akinesia of the mid–free wall with preserved apical contractility (McConnell sign) (**Fig. 7**A), flattening of the interventricular septum in systole (D shape of the left ventricle) (**Fig. 7**B), and moderate tricuspid regurgitation with Doppler-derived pulmonary artery systolic pressure, 65 mm Hg (**Fig. 7**C, D). Echogenic masses were noted at the level of proximal right and left pulmonary arteries (**Fig. 7**E). A dilated inferior vena cava was observed (**Fig. 7** F). CTPA confirmed extensive bilateral pulmonary arteries filling defects extending to bilateral lobar and segmental branches in keeping with PE (**Fig. 8**A, B) and flattening of the interventricular septum (**Fig. 8**C), suggestive of right ventricular strain. The patient was put on rivaroxaban, 15 mg twice a day for 21 days followed by 20 mg once daily. She was not suitable for recombinant tissue plasminogen activator because she had had a recent spinal cord surgery. She was discharged after 2 weeks in good clinical condition without need of supplement oxygen. Three months later, on follow-up TTE there was complete recovery of the right ventricular dimension and function and trivial tricuspid regurgitation without increase in pulmonary pressure (**Fig. 9**).

Acute Aortic Dissection

Classical acute aortic dissection (AAD) (80%–90% of acute aortic syndromes; incidence from 2.6 per 100,000 to 3.5 cases per 100,000 person-years) represents life-treating clinical entity affecting the aorta media layer and characterized by the presence of an intimal flap separating the true and false lumens (double-barrel appearance).[25] Due to the clinical presentation heterogeneity, the diagnosis may be challenging, with substantial delay in

timely and appropriate therapeutic interventions and consequent negative impact on outcome. Anatomically it is commonly classified (Stanford system) into 2 categories regardless of the site of origin: type A involves the ascending aorta, and type B does not involve the ascending aorta. Open surgery is the recommended treatment of type A AAD (in-hospital mortality approximately 22%). On the other hand, medical therapy alone is the treatment of choice for uncomplicated type B AAD (in-hospital mortality approximately 11%). Thoracic endovascular aortic repair currently is recommended only for complicated type B AAD.[25]

Clinical case: type A acute aortic dissection

A 40-year-old woman presented to the ED complaining during the previous 6 weeks of on-off tearing chest pain radiating to the back and neck. Past medical history consisted of history of systemic lupus erythromatosus, end-stage renal disease (glomerular filtration rate, 14 mL/min), systemic hypertension, and gout. On physical examination (HR, 87 BPM, and BP, 148/89 mm Hg), an early diastolic murmur (4/6) on aortic area was heard. No pulse deficits detected. Laboratory test were as follows: Hb, 7.8 g/L; creatinine, 439 umol/L; potassium, 4.9 mmol/L; and troponin, negative. ECG and CXR were unremarkable (**Fig. 10**). TTE was performed to rule out wall motion abnormalities and showed type A aortic dissection (**Fig. 11**A-D) confirmed by TEE (**Fig. 11**E–G) and CT (**Fig. 12**). The patient underwent ascending aortic replacement along with resuspension of aortic valve and false lumen obliteration (**Fig. 13**). The patient was discharged after 10 days without any major complication. Clinical and imaging (CT) follow-up was scheduled at 1 months.

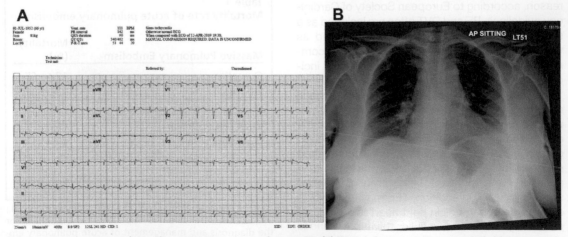

Fig. 6. (*A*) ECG, sinus tachycardia. S1Q3T3 pattern of acute PE. (*B*) CXR, left costophrenic angle is blunted. Right costophrenic angle is clear.

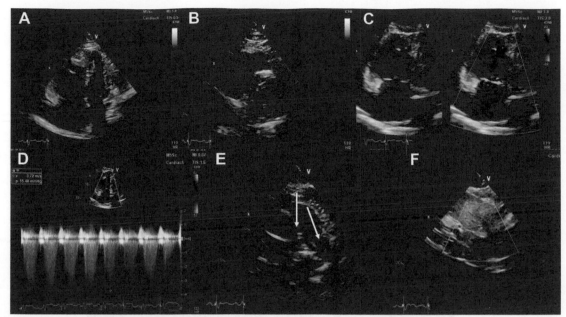

Fig. 7. TTE in the ER. (*A*) Short axis with D-shape of interventricular septum, particularly in systole. (*B*) Four-chamber view showing the right ventricle dilated and bigger than the left ventricle. (*C*) Acceleration time on right ventricular outflow tract of 50 ms. (*D*) Tricuspid regurgitation Doppler signal showing dense and triangular Doppler signal with peak gradient of 55 mm Hg. (*E*) Short axis on the grate vessels. The arrows indicate the thrombus in the left and right pulmonary artery. (*F*) Dilated inferior vena cava.

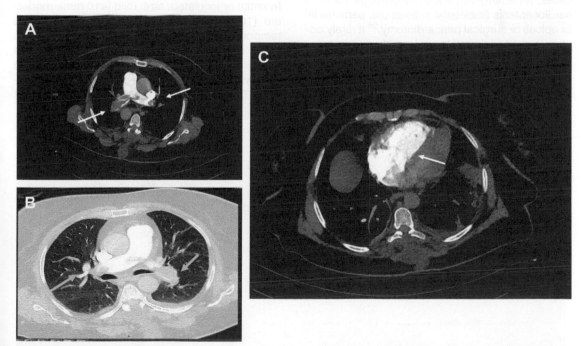

Fig. 8. Chest CT. (*A*) and (*B*) Extensive bilateral pulmonary arteries filling defects extending to bilateral lobar and segmental branches (*white and green arrows*) in keeping with acute PE. (*A*) Mediastinal window. (*B*) Pulmonary window. (*C*) There is flattening of the interventricular septum (*white arrow*) suggestive of right ventricular strain without any signs of pulmonary hypertension. Minimal left pleural effusion with adjacent atelectasis.

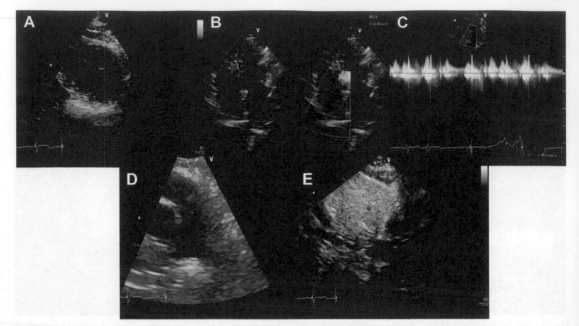

Fig. 9. (*A*) No D-shape of the left ventricle. (*B*) Right ventricle is not dilated. (*C*) No significant tricuspid regurgitation. (*D*) No thrombus seen in the pulmonary arteries. (*E*) Normal inferior vena cava.

Cardiac Tamponade

Cardiac tamponade (incidence, 5 cases per 10,000 ED admissions) represents a life-threatening clinical entity needing, in a majority of cases, an emergent pericardial drainage via pericardiocentesis (subcostal/subxiphoid, parasternal or apical) or surgical pericardiotomy.[26] It rarely occurs in acute idiopathic pericarditis and is more common in patients with a specific underlying etiology, such as malignancy (52%), idiopathic condition (14.6%), end-stage renal kidney disease (12.5%), iatrogenic disease (7.3%), and infective diseases (2.1%, tubercolosis or purulent pericarditis).[27] It is important to underline that clinically significant tamponade depends not only on the size of pericardial effusion but also on the rapidity with which the fluid is formed (distribution: circumferential or loculated; size: mild [<10 mm], moderate [10–20 mm], or large [>20 mm]). Cardiac tamponade is defined as acute when it occurs within minutes, usually due to trauma or rupture of the heart or aorta or as a complication of an invasive diagnostic and/or therapeutic procedures. The clinical picture consists of cardiogenic

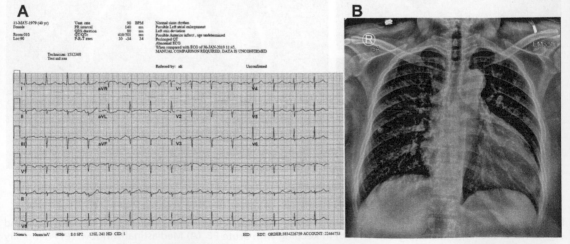

Fig. 10. (*A*) ECG, sinus rhythm. (*B*) CXR, mild to moderate cardiomegaly with prominence of the pulmonary vasculature. No other significant interval changes are seen.

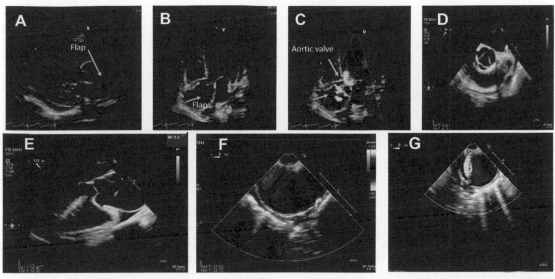

Fig. 11. (*A*) Long axis, dissection flap (*yellow arrow*) on the ascending aorta at the level of the sinotubular junction: small pericardial effusion. (*B*) Five-chamber view. The dissection flap is seen below the aortic valve (*arrow*). (*C*) With color, the convergence flow is seen at the level of the flap (*yellow arrow*). The green arrow indicates the aortic valve. (*D*) Parasternal short axis view at the level of the great vessels. TEE in (*E*), (*F*) and (*G*) flap of the ascending aorta at 120°, aortic arch and descending aorta.

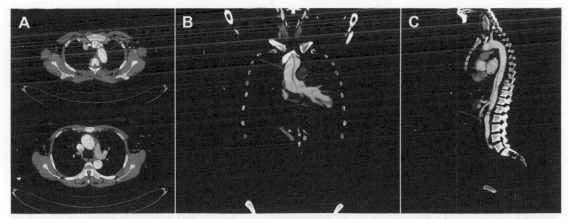

Fig. 12. (*A*) Transverse view; arrows indicate the dissection at the level of the ascending aorta and arch. (*B*) Coronal view; the dissection (*arrow*) is just above the aortic valve. (*C*) Sagittal view; the dissection (*arrow*) reaches the iliac arteries.

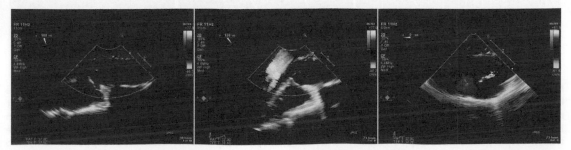

Fig. 13. TEE postsurgery. The images showed false lumen obliteration and mild residual aortic regurgitation.

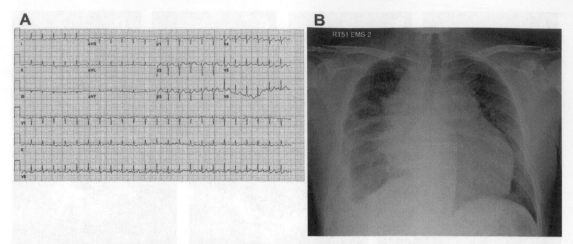

Fig. 14. (A) ECG, HR approximately 143 BPM. Nonspecific ST and T-wave changes. (B) CXR, a wide mediastinum with increased cardiac silhouette, right pleural effusion, and pulmonary edema.

shock requiring urgent reduction in pericardial pressure. On the other hand, subacute/chronic occurs over days to weeks. However, the patients may be asymptomatic until intrapericardial pressure reaches a critical value. Echocardiography is the method of choice for diagnosis, because it defines the severity of tamponade and enables safer and reliable percutaneous drainage compared with a blind approach.[28,29]

Clinical case: tamponade in Hodgkin lymphoma
A 45-year-old male patient, known to have mediastinal Hodgkin lymphoma underwent and failed multiple chemotherapeutic treatment regimens. He presented to the ED with dyspnea on minimal exertion, chest discomfort, lower limb edema, and easy fatigability. He was tachycardic and hypotensive (HR, 125 BPM, and BP, 80/40 mm Hg), his neck veins were dilated, and he had lower

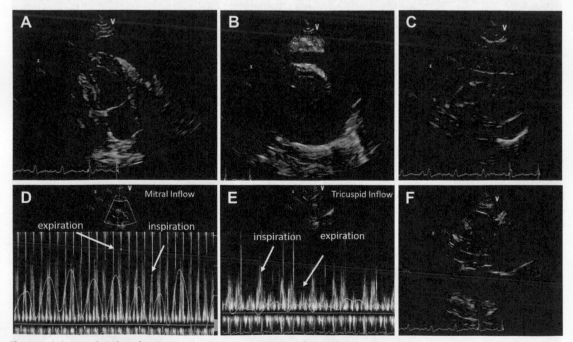

Fig. 15. (A) Apical 4-chamber view revealed a large pericardial effusion. (B) Parasternal short axis view revealed a large circumferential pericardial effusion. (C) Subcostal view revealed a large pericardial effusion with diastolic right ventricular collapse. (D) Respiratory variation in the transmitral pulse-wave Doppler: inspiratory reduction in mitral peak E-wave velocity in cardiac tamponade will drop of at least 25%. (E) Respiratory variation in the transtricuspid pulsed-wave Doppler: the tricuspid peak E-wave velocity drops at least 40% in expiration compared with inspiration. (F) Dilated and noncollapsible inferior vena cava.

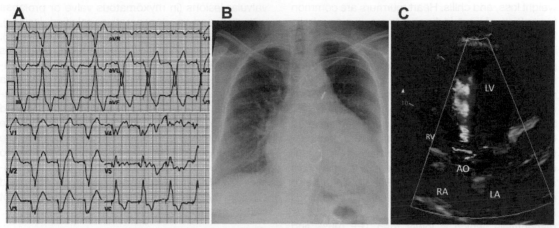

Fig. 16. (*A*) ECG. (*B*) CXR. (*C*) TTE with color doppler, 5 chamber view; severe aortic regurgitation. AO, aorta; LA, left atrium; LV, left ventricle; RA, right atrium; RV right ventricle.

limbs edema up to his knees. ECG showed sinus tachycardia with low voltage in the peripheral leads, and CXR showed wide mediastinum with increased cardiac silhouette, right pleural effusion, and pulmonary edema (**Fig. 14**). TTE (**Fig. 15**A–F) was performed and showed large pericardial effusion, collapsed right ventricle, significant respiratory variation in the transmitral pulsed-wave Doppler, and dilated and noncollapsible inferior vena cava. He underwent an ultrasound-guided pericardiocentesis, apical approach; 500 mL of a cloudy, turbid, and serous pericardial fluid was aspirated. The patient was admitted to the hospital and his symptoms improved. The pericardial fluid cytology analysis revealed atypical cells consistent with Hodgkin lymphoma.

Infective Endocarditis

In developed countries, the incidence of infective endocarditis (IE) ranges from 2 cases per 100,000 to 11.6 cases per 100,000 patients/y and is higher in urban than rural settings, reflecting drug use. In developed countries, mitral prolapse and degenerative cardiac lesions are the common predisposing lesions, whereas in developing countries, rheumatic heart disease remain the leading disease. Mortality ranges from 16% to 27%, higher in those with severe comorbid illness. Most common organism is methicillin-resistant *Staphylococcus aureus*.[30,31]

The clinical history of IE is extremely variable, including its presentation; therefore, it easily may mislead an initial assessment.[1] It can vary from an acute (rapidly progressive infection) to a subacute or chronic disease characterized by nonspecific symptoms and signs (low-grade fever). Up to 90% of patients present with fever associated with systemic symptoms, including poor appetite,

Box 2 Echocardiographic characteristics of endocarditis lesions	
Vegetation	Flickering mass or nonoscillating intracardiac mass on valve or other endocardial structures or on implanted intracardiac material
Abscess	Thickened, nonhomogeneous perivalvular area with echodense or echolucent appearance
Pseudoaneurysm	Pulsatile perivalvular echo-free space, with color Doppler flow detected
Perforation	Interruption of endocardial tissue
Fistula	Color Doppler communication between 2 neighboring cavities through a perforation.
Valve aneurysm	Saccular bulging of valvular tissue.
Dehiscence of a prosthetic valve	Paravalvular regurgitation identified by TTE/TEE, with or without rocking motion of the prosthesis.

Data from Refs.[30–34]

weight loss, and chills. Heart murmurs are common (up to 85% of IE); 1 in 4 patients may have embolic fearsome complications at presentation (to the brain, lung, spleen, or kidney). Classic signs and peripheral stigmata of IE also include vascular and immunologic phenomena, such as splinter hemorrhages, Roth spots, and glomerulonephritis. Diagnostic suspicion may be strengthened by laboratory signs of infection, such as elevated CRP or erythrocyte sedimentation rate, leukocytosis, anemia, and microscopic hematuria. Echocardiography plays a pivotal role in both diagnosis and management of IE.[30–33] TTE is the first choice method, with sensitivity for diagnosis of vegetations in native and prosthetic valves of 70% and 50%, respectively, which is lower than TEE (96% and 92%, respectively).[34] Moreover, the implementation of the 3-dimensional (3-D) modality increases the accuracy of TEE further, especially for mitral valve IE. In any case, the identification of vegetations can be difficult in the presence of preexisting valvular lesions (in myxomatous valve or prolapse with flail and in degenerative calcified lesions), prosthetic valves, small vegetations (2–3 mm), recent embolization, and nonvegetant IE. Diagnosis may be challenging, particularly in IE affecting intracardiac devices, even with the use of TEE. As a general rule, if the TTE/TEE is negative with low suspicion of IE, no other investigation is needed (**Box 2**). On the other hand, if TTE/TEE is negative but there is still a high IE clinical suspicion, the exams should to be repeated after 7 days to 10 days. Other imaging techniques, such as multislice CT, MRI, ^{18}F-fluorodeoxyglucose PET, and CT, may help in the final diagnosis[1,3,4] but are not part of the ED diagnostic tools.[32,33]

Clinical case: aortic valve perforation

A 45-year-old woman presented to the ED with a 1-month history of shortness of breath and fever. Two years earlier she underwent mitral mechanical valve replacement and tricuspid valve repair

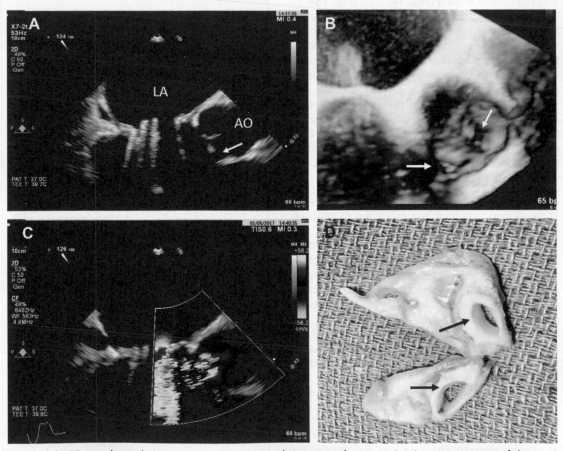

Fig. 17. (*A*) TEE, esophageal view at 120°. The arrow points to a perforation of right coronary cusp of the aortic valve. (*B*) 3-D echocardiography, anatomic view of the aortic valve showing a perforation of the right and left coronary cusps (*white arrows*). (*C*) TEE color Doppler, severe aortic regurgitation; 2 regurgitant jets. (*D*) Anatomic specimen, perforation of right and left coronary cusps (*black arrows*). AO, aorta; LA, left atrium.

(annuloplasty ring) along with pacemaker implantation. She was alert, oriented, and febrile (37.8°C). Physical examination revealed tachycardia and holodiastolic murmur on aorta valve area. From the laboratory results, she had increased inflammatory parameters (CRP = 5.9 mg/L); ECG rhythm related to pacemaker; and, on the CXR, a mechanical valve in mitral position and the leads of the PM were seen (**Fig. 16**). TTE was performed and showed severe aortic regurgitation with left ventricular dilatation and normal systolic function (see **Fig. 16**C). The TEE revealed the perforation of 2 cusps of the aortic valve with severe aortic regurgitation (**Fig. 17**A–C) that was confirmed at surgery (**Fig. 17**D).

SUMMARY

A simple stepwise biomarker imaging evaluation of several CVEs is described that the authors hope is beneficial in making rapid diagnosis of these conditions in the ED and thus help in timely treatment and improved outcomes of these patients.

DISCLOSURE

The authors have nothing to disclose.

REFERENCES

1. Benjiamin EJ, Muntner P, Alonso A, et al. Heart Disease and Stroke Statistics— 2019 Update. A Report From the American Heart Association. Circulation 2019;139:e56–528.
2. Neskovic NA, Hagendorff A, Lancellotti L, et al. on behalf of the European Association of Cardiovascular Imaging. Emergency echocardiography: the European Association of Cardiovascular Imaging recommendations. Eur Heart J Cardiovasc Imaging 2013;14:1–11.
3. Suzuki T, Lyon A, Saggar R, et al. Editor's Choice-Biomarkers of acute cardiovascular and pulmonary diseases. Eur Heart J Acute Cardiovasc Care 2016;5(5):416–33.
4. Dobra M, Bordi L, Nyulas T, et al. Computed Tomography — an Emerging Tool for Triple Rule-Out in the Emergency Department. A Review. J Cardiovasc Emerg 2017;3(1):36–40.
5. Dastidar AG, Baritussio A, De Garate E, et al. Prognostic Role of CMR and Conventional Risk Factors in Myocardial Infarction With Nonobstructed Coronary Arteries. JACC Cardiovasc Imaging 2019;12(10):1973–82.
6. Ibanez B, James S, Agewall S, et al, ESC Scientific Document Group. 2017 ESC Guidelines for the management of acute myocardial infarction in patients presenting with ST-segment elevation: The Task Force for the management of acute myocardial infarction in patients presenting with ST-segment elevation of the European Society of Cardiology (ESC). Eur Heart J 2018;39(2):119–77.
7. Weinsaft JW, Kim RJ, Ross M, et al. Contrast-enhanced anatomic imaging as compared to contrast-enhanced tissue characterization for detection of left ventricular thrombus. JACC Cardiovasc Imaging 2009;2(8):969–79.
8. Konstantinides SV, Meyer G, Becattini C, et al, ESC Scientific Document Group. 2019 ESC Guidelines for the diagnosis and management of acute pulmonary embolism developed in collaboration with the European Respiratory Society (ERS). Eur Heart J 2020;41(4):543–603.
9. Thygensen K, Alpert J, Jaffe AS, et al. Fourth universal definition of myocardial infarction (2018). Eur Heart J 2019;40:237–69.
10. Hamm CW, Bassand JP, Agewall S, et al, ESC Committee for Practice Guidelines. ESC Guidelines for the management of acute coronary syndromes in patients presenting without persistent ST-segment elevation: The Task Force for the management of acute coronary syndromes (ACS) in patients presenting without persistent ST-segment elevation of the European Society of Cardiology (ESC). Eur Heart J 2011;32(23):2999–3054.
11. Kully R, Jones N, Moorianj N. Mechanical Complications of Acute Myocardial Infarction. Cardiol Clin 2013;31:519–31.
12. Evrin T, Unluer EE, Kuday E, et al. Bedside Echocardiography in Acute Myocardial Infarction Patients with Hemodynamic Deterioration. J Natl Med Assoc 2018;110(4):396–8.
13. Bahit MC, Kochar A, Granger BG, et al. Post-Myocardial Infarction Heart Failure. JACC Heart Fail 2018;6:179–86.
14. Yip H, Wu C, Chang H, et al. Cardiac rupture complicating acute myocardial infarction in the direct percutaneous coronary intervention reperfusion era. Chest 2003;124:561–71.
15. Ghadri JR, Wittstein IS, Prasad A, et al. International Expert Consensus Document on Takotsubo Syndrome (Part I): Clinical Characteristics, Diagnostic Criteria, and Pathophysiology. Eur Heart J 2018;39:2032–46.
16. Ghadri JR, Wittstein IS, Prasad A, et al. International Expert Consensus Document on Takotsubo Syndrome (Part II): Diagnostic Workup, Outcome, and Management. Eur Heart J 2018;39:2047–62.
17. Lyon AR, Bossone E, Schneider B, et al. Current state of knowledge on Takotsubo syndrome: a Position Statement from the Taskforce on Takotsubo Syndrome of the Heart Failure Association of the European Society of Cardiology. Eur J Heart Fail 2016;18(1):8–27.
18. Citro R, Rigo F, D'Andrea A, et al. Echocardiographic correlates of acute heart failure, cardiogenic shock, and in-hospital mortality in tako-tsubo

cardiomyopathy. JACC Cardiovasc Imaging 2014;7: 119–29.

19. Bossone E, Lyon A, Citro R, et al. Takotsubo cardiomyopathy: an integrated multi-imaging approach. Eur Heart J Cardiovasc Imaging 2014;15(4):366–77.

20. Caforio AL, Pankuweit S, Arbustini E, et al, European Society of Cardiology Working Group on Myocardial and Pericardial Diseases. Current state of knowledge on aetiology, diagnosis, management, and therapy of myocarditis: a position statement of the European Society of Cardiology Working Group on Myocardial and Pericardial Diseases. Eur Heart J 2013;34(33):2636–48, 2648a-2648d.

21. Pollack A, Kontorovich AR, Fuster V, et al. Viral myocarditis–diagnosis, treatment options, and current controversies. Nat Rev Cardiol 2015;12(11): 670–80.

22. Hritani R, Alrifai A, Soud M, et al. Which patients with pulmonary embolism need echocardiography? Cleve Clin J Med 2018;85(11):826–8.

23. Cohen R, Loarte P, Navarro V, et al. Echocardiographic findings in pulmonary embolism: An important guide for the management of the patient. World J Cardiovasc Dis 2012;2:161–4.

24. Stein PD, Fowler SE, Goodman LR, et al, PIOPED II Investigators. Multidetector computed tomography after acute pulmonary embolism. N Engl J Med 2006;354:2317–27.

25. Erbel R, Aboyans V, Boileau C, et al, ESC Committee for Practice Guidelines. 2014 ESC Guidelines on the diagnosis and treatment of aortic diseases: Document covering acute and chronic aortic diseases of the thoracic and abdominal aorta of the adult. The Task Force for the Diagnosis and Treatment of Aortic Diseases of the European Society of Cardiology (ESC). Eur Heart J 2014;35(41): 2873–926.

26. Adler Y, Charron P, Imazio M, et al. 2015 ESC Guidelines for the diagnosis and management of pericardial diseases: The Task Force for the Diagnosis and Management of Pericardial Diseases of the European Society of Cardiology (ESC)Endorsed by: The European Association for Cardio-Thoracic Surgery (EACTS). Eur Heart J 2015;36:2921.

27. Navarrete OC, Ortuño F, Rocamora J, et al. Should we try to determine the specific cause of cardiac tamponade? Rev Esp Cardiol 2002;55(5):493–8.

28. Imazio M, Adler Y. Management of pericardial effusion. Eur Heart J 2013;34(16):1186–97.

29. Tsang TS, Freeman WK, Barnes ME, et al. Rescue echocardiographically guided pericardiocentesis for cardiac perforation complicating catheter-based procedures. The Mayo Clinic experience. J Am Coll Cardiol 1998;32:1345.

30. Habib G, Lancellotti P, Antunes MJ, et al. ESC Scientific Document Group, 2015 ESC Guidelines for the management of infective endocarditis: The Task Force for the Management of Infective Endocarditis of the European Society of Cardiology (ESC) Endorsed by: European Association for Cardio-Thoracic Surgery (EACTS), the European Association of Nuclear Medicine (EANM). Eur Heart J 2015;36:3075–128.

31. Habib G. How do we reduce embolic risk and mortality in infective endocarditis? Measure the size of the vegetation and operate early in patients with large vegetations. Eur Heart J 2019;40(27):2252–4.

32. Afonso L, Kottam A, Reddy V, et al. Echocardiography in infective endocarditis: state of the art. Curr Cardiol Rep 2017;19:127.

33. Cahill TH, Baddour LM, Habib G, et al. Challenges in infective endocarditis. J Am Coll Cardiol 2017;69: 325–44.

34. Schauer SG, Pfaff JA, Cuenca PJ. Emergency department management of acute infective endocarditis. Emerg Med Pract 2014;16(11):1–17 [quiz: 17-8].

Clinical Application of Stress Echocardiography in Management of Heart Failure

Kenya Kusunose, MD, PhD

KEYWORDS

- Cardiac output • Left ventricular filling pressure • Heart failure • Tricuspid regurgitation
- Transmitral flow • Stress echocardiography • Preload stress

KEY POINTS

- Filling pressures and cardiac output can change dynamically during stress. Thus, we are unable to decide the accurate state in heart failure (HF) at resting at a single time point.
- The key to understanding hemodynamics in HF is the relation between elevated left ventricular (LV) filling pressure and cardiac output.
- Physiologic stress methods can be widely applied to acquire comprehensive hemodynamic data and images at rest and subsequently at peak levels.
- Recently, preload stress echocardiography using leg lifting or leg-positive pressure maneuver was reported to noninvasively reproduce volume central shift without any increase in total body fluid volume.
- E/e' and estimated systolic pulmonary artery pressure are "relatively" good markers of LV filling pressure even in the modern era.

 Video content accompanies this article at http://www.heartfailure.theclinics.com.

INTRODUCTION

Heart failure (HF) is the most common cause of death in cardiovascular disease.[1,2] The incidence of HF continues to increase in aging populations. For the management of HF, precise evaluation of disease severity and prediction of adverse outcome are crucial.[3] Several reports have shown that diastolic function plays an important role in HF.[4] Left ventricular (LV) filling pressure and cardiac output, common pathways affecting LV diastolic function, are considered to be important diagnostic targets that should be measured or estimated at rest and during stress.[5] Although there are exertional limitations in HF patients, resting cardiac filling pressures are often normal, and cardiac outputs are also normal. LV filling pressures and cardiac output can change dynamically during stress loading in patients with confirmed or suspected HF. Thus, we are unable to decide the accurate state of HF at a resting single time point. To overcome this issue, stress echocardiography should be applied for hemodynamic assessment.

The key to hemodynamics in HF is a balance of elevated LV filling pressure and cardiac output. Patients with HF often show diastolic dysfunction with impaired active LV relaxation and passive LV chamber stiffness.[6] Patients with grade I

Funding: The author has no funding to disclose.
Ethical Statements: All procedures followed were in accordance with the ethical standards of the responsible committee on human experimentation (institutional and national) and with the Helsinki Declaration of 1964 and later versions.
Department of Cardiovascular Medicine, Tokushima University Hospital, 2-50-1 Kuramoto, Tokushima, Japan
E-mail address: kusunosek@tokushima-u.ac.jp

Heart Failure Clin 16 (2020) 347–355
https://doi.org/10.1016/j.hfc.2020.02.001
1551-7136/20/© 2020 Elsevier Inc. All rights reserved.

diastolic dysfunction have normal LV filling pressure at rest. However, some patients show abnormal response to stress in the relationship between LV filling pressure and cardiac output. In patients with preserved diastolic function, cardiac output can be increased without significantly elevated filling pressure during stress. In patients with HF, as long as the Frank-Starling mechanism operates effectively, cardiac output can increase at the expense of elevated filling pressure. In patients with decompensated HF, hemodynamic stress will lead to a much greater elevation in filling pressure, pulmonary venous hypertension, and subsequent pulmonary congestion without an effective increase in cardiac output (**Fig. 1**). Based on this phenomenon, stress echocardiography may be beneficial in identifying the accurate state of HF and risk of adverse outcome.

Stress echocardiography is widely used to assess several cardiovascular diseases, including ischemic heart disease, valvular heart disease (VHD), HF, congenital heart disease, and pulmonary hypertension.[7–12] In this review, the authors focus on the current and future directions regarding the use of stress echocardiography in HF.

MEASUREMENTS DURING EXERCISE

Physiologic stress methods can be widely applied to acquire comprehensive hemodynamic data and images at rest and subsequently at peak levels. The advantages and disadvantages between different techniques in stress echocardiography are shown in **Table 1**. Physiologic stress is mainly performed by 6 types of application.[13]

In the treadmill test, the Bruce protocol or modified Bruce protocol is used.[14] After exercise, it is critical to complete postexercise imaging as quickly as possible because hemodynamic and echocardiographic parameters normalize rapidly

during recovery. The 6-minute walk test is widely available to assess exercise capacity and prognosis in several cardiovascular and pulmonary diseases. This test is similar to treadmill stress, and imaging should be performed after exercise as soon as possible.

In bicycle ergometer stress echocardiography, the patient pedals through a workload that is increased in a stepwise manner (25 W/2–3 minutes) while imaging is performed. The advantage of a semisupine bicycle is the availability of image acquisition during stress. At peak stress, cardiac function in HF can be assessed appropriately. In addition, with the patient in the supine position, it is easy to acquire images from multiple views during stress. Maximum workload is slightly lower in the supine bicycle stress compared with conventional treadmill stress; however, the workload is sufficient enough to assess HF.

Recently, preload stress echocardiography using leg lifting or leg-positive pressure maneuver (**Fig. 2**) was reported to noninvasively reproduce volume central shift without any increase in total body fluid volume, thus, disclosing the preload reserve for patients with chronic HF.[15–19] Leg-positive pressure maneuver is designed to provide a continuous external pressure around both lower limbs using specialized airbags at 90-mm Hg pressure (Video 1). This pressure safely provides an effective increase in ventricular preload with evidence based on the findings from invasive hemodynamic studies.[20,21] Echocardiographic measurements were obtained both at rest and during stress. Acquiring images were performed 20 seconds after the inflation of the airbags. If the data acquisition time elapsed greater than 3 minutes, airbags were temporarily deflated and then reinflated to ensure that leg-positive pressure stress could continue to provide adequate preload stress. Leg-positive pressure is contraindicated in

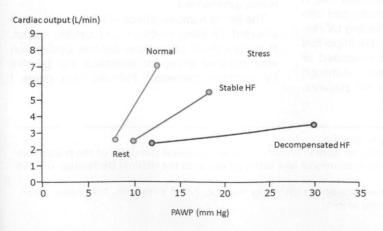

Cardiac output (L/min)

Fig. 1. Comparison of CO and PAWP based on hypothetical data. The key to understanding hemodynamics in HF is the relation between elevated LV filling pressure and cardiac output. The relationship between CO and PAWP in 3 types of cohorts (normal, stable heart failure, and decompensated HF).

Table 1
Comparison of advantages and disadvantages between different techniques in stress echocardiography

Methods	Allows for Imaging at Peak Levels	Assessment During Stress	Quantitative Assessment	Ischemic Assessment	Availability	Risk of Complication
Ergometer	No	No	Strong	Strong	Low	Low
Treadmill	Yes	Yes	Strong	Strong	Moderate	Low
6-min walk test	No	No	Weak	Weak	High	Low
Leg-positive pressure	Yes	Yes	Modest	No	Very low	Very low
Leg lifting	Yes	Yes	Weak	No	High	Very low
Hand grip	Yes	Yes	Weak	Weak	Moderate	Very low

patients with a history of venous thrombosis/pulmonary embolism, or severe orthopedic traumatic disease and active skin lesions in the lower limbs.

The hand grip test is a simple tool that increases LV afterload and myocardial oxygen demand without respiratory artifacts.[22] Handgrip exercise has long been used during invasive assessment of LV filling pressures, providing differentiation between several patient groups, including those at risk for or with established HF. In general, 3 minutes of handgrip exercise is performed at 40% of maximum grip strength, determined before baseline imaging. All clinical and echocardiographic data were recorded during the final minute of isometric handgrip exercise.

MEASUREMENTS DURING EXERCISE

In HF, pulmonary arterial wedge pressures (PAWP; a surrogate marker of left atrial pressure) during stress exceed those in general cohorts. In this regard, PAWP during exercise can aid in HF

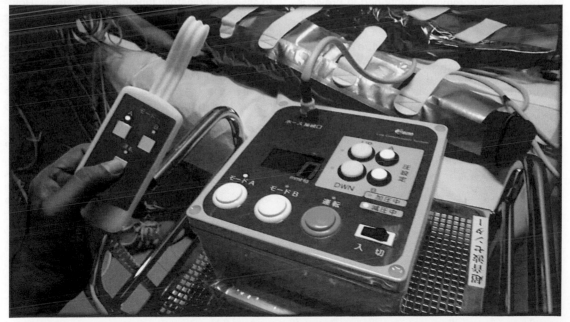

Fig. 2. Preload stress echocardiography using leg-positive pressure. Preload stress echocardiography using leg-positive pressure maneuver (Corona Leg Compression System; Corona Industries Ltd, Yoshinogawa, Japan) was reported to noninvasively reproduce volume central shift without any increase in total body fluid volume.

diagnosis. Moreover, it has been used to define inclusion criteria for clinical trials in both HF with preserved EF and reduced EF.

Based on the Frank-Starling mechanisms, increased cardiac output during stress is coupled with elevation of PAWP. Evaluation of PAWP during stress in the absence of knowledge about cardiac output may be problematic. Several investigators showed that the relationship between PAWP and cardiac output might be crucial in assessing the stage of HF. From 4 recently published studies using exercise right heart catheter data, the scatter plots seem to be categorized into 3 components (**Fig. 3**).[19,23–26] In stage A HF (at risk, control group), cardiac output easily increases with slight elevation of PAWP during stress. Δ cardiac output (CO)/ΔPAWP is around 0.8 to 1.0.[23–25] In patients with stage B HF (mild diastolic dysfunction), cardiac output can increase at the expense of elevated PAWP. ΔCO/ΔPAWP is around 0.4 to 0.6.[23,24] In stages C and D HF (severe diastolic dysfunction including heart failure reduced ejection fraction [HFrEF]), stress test will lead to significant elevation in PAWP with only slightly increased cardiac output. ΔCO/ΔPAWP is around 0.1 to 0.2.[19,25,26] According to these studies, the optimal cutoff value of ΔCO/ΔPAWP to find severely impaired LV diastolic function is around 0.3. Both cardiac output and PAWP should be assessed in suspected or confirmed HF.

In stress echocardiography, the parameter that has been most commonly mentioned in previous studies is the E/e′ ratio. E/e′ was previously validated as a marker of mean PAWP during stress.[27,28] In the original paper, E/e′ has been found to correlate well to mean PAWP through Nagueh's formula: PCWP = 1.9 + 1.24(E/e′).[29] Even if there are technical challenges and problems of accuracy in measuring E and e′, such as

instances of increased heart rate and cases with A wave fused to E wave during stress, this index is widely used in many laboratories. Increased E/e′ during stress is not specific in the assessment of HF, because it may be caused by ischemia, pulmonary arterial hypertension (chamber interaction), or other cardiac/noncardiac diseases. E/e′ may also be misleading in cases of mitral annular calcification, moderate to severe mitral regurgitation, constrictive pericarditis, mitral valve repair or replacement, left bundle branch block, or significant aortic regurgitation.[30]

Systolic pulmonary artery pressure (sPAP) is a key marker of right ventricular function used to assess LV diastolic function. The estimation of sPAP is based on the tricuspid regurgitation (TR) pressure gradient by simplified Bernoulli equation, which takes into account estimated right atrial pressure in the absence of right ventricular outflow tract obstruction. An increase in sPAP after stress has been reported to be correlated with increases in the LV filling pressures, recorded by invasive measurements.[28]

E/e′ and sPAP are not perfect markers to estimate changes in LV filling pressure; thus, more appropriate methods are desired. Some other stress echocardiographic variables to be recorded have been described in previous reports.[31] Instead of E/e′, other variables, such as suction (flow propagation velocity), relaxation (isovolumic relaxation time and deceleration time), and compliance (A duration and pulmonary venous flow) are tested to assess LV diastolic function during stress. However, because these markers have the problem of availability and reproducibility, E/e′ and sPAP are still "relatively" good markers of LV filling pressure even in the modern era.

Doppler-derived cardiac output is frequently observed in the clinical setting. Several studies showed a good correlation between cardiac

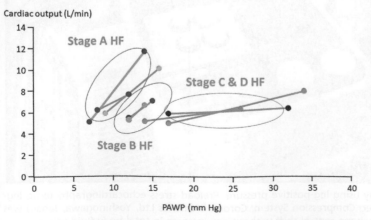

Fig. 3. Comparison of CO and PAWP based on previous invasive studies. Several investigators showed that the relation between PAWP and cardiac output might be more likely to assess the stage of HF.

outputs calculated by Doppler echocardiography and invasive thermodilution and Fick methods.[32,33] On the other hand, in treadmill test and 6-minute walk test, it is difficult to measure the 2 important measurements (PAWP and cardiac output) at the same peak level. To overcome this issue, electrical cardiometry can be used to measure the cardiac output at the same time as echocardiogram.[34] This method was also validated in previous studies.[35]

EXERCISE STRESS ECHOCARDIOGRAPHY FOR HEART FAILURE

Exercise stress echocardiography has been developed to detect exercise-induced changes of hemodynamic parameters (eg, increase in LV filling pressures) assessed by Doppler echocardiography during exercise. Echocardiographic parameters during exercise can assess not only the diagnosis but also therapeutic effects. A randomized study conducted in heart failure preserved ejection fraction patients showed a 58% reduction of the exercise-induced increase in estimated LV filling pressure, after short-term treatment with ivabradine compared with placebo. Exercise capacity also improved after the treatment. Interestingly, changes in E/e' correlated with changes in exercise capacity.[36] A nonrandomized study in suspected pulmonary

hypertension patients also showed a decrease in exercise-induced impairment of pulmonary vascular capacity, after pulmonary artery hypertension-specific therapy.[23]

REPRESENTATIVE CASES USING EXERCISE ECHOCARDIOGRAPHY

The first case is a woman in her 60s. She was referred to the author's hospital with a history of hypertension (**Fig. 4**). She noted fatigue in daily activities. LV ejection fraction was preserved. Regional wall motion abnormality was not detected. Transmitral flow E and A waves were similar height, and TR velocity (TR-V) was around 2.5 m per second. Pulmonary hypertension was not detected at baseline. At peak stress, LV inflow significantly increased and E/e' also increased from 8 to 15 (estimated PCWP from 12 to 21). Estimated pulmonary artery pressure significantly increased from 37 to 60 mm Hg. Cardiac output also increased from 4.0 L/min to 6.0 L/min. Thus, ΔCO/ΔPCWP was 0.2. This patient had exercise-induced elevated LV filling pressure/pulmonary hypertension and severely impaired LV.

The second case is a man in his 70s. He was referred to the author's hospital with a history of diabetes mellitus (**Fig. 5**). LV ejection fraction was preserved. Regional wall motion abnormality

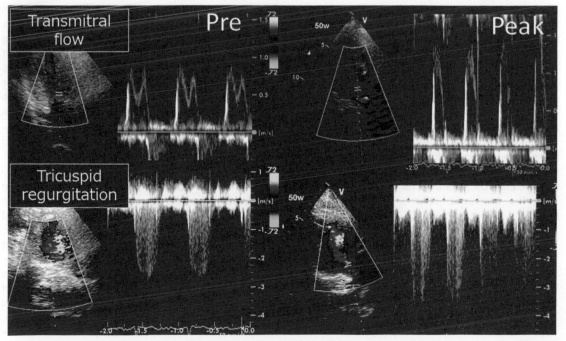

Fig. 4. A case with ergometer stress. The patient had exercise-induced elevated LV filling pressure and pulmonary hypertension.

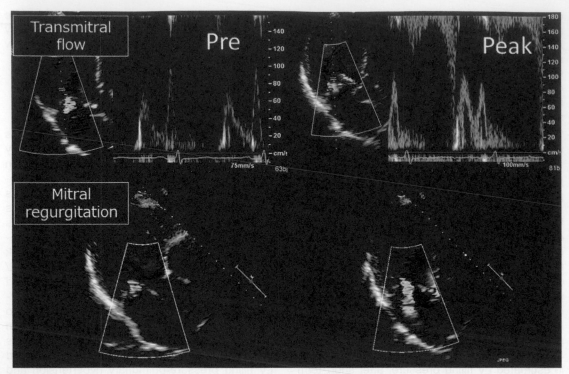

Fig. 5. A case with handgrip stress. The patient had exercise-induced elevated LV filling pressure and mitral regurgitation.

was not detected. In this case, hand grip at 50% maximum effort was applied. During hand grip stress, E wave increased and A wave decreased. Mitral regurgitation significantly increased during hand grip stress. Thus, the author's group diagnosed the patient with exercise-induced elevated LV filling pressure and mitral regurgitation.

PRELOAD STRESS ECHOCARDIOGRAPHY FOR HEART FAILURE

An important factor of cardiac reserve is the ability to enhance cardiac output without significantly increasing ventricular filling pressure, in response to increased venous return. Thus, the preload reserve can be regarded as a representative of both the contractile reserve and the diastolic reserve.

As a simplified method of increasing preload, previous investigators performed passive leg-lifting maneuvers. They reported that this technique could be used to assess functional reserve in patients with HF. Pozzoli and colleagues[37] and Ishizu and colleagues[38] performed passive leg-lifting maneuvers on HF patients who showed an impaired relaxation pattern of LV inflow at baseline. They evaluated diastolic reserve by using passive leg lifting. Patients who showed the

inverted E/A ratio during leg lifting had an occult diastolic dysfunction despite having normal LV filling pressure at baseline. Abe and colleagues[39] also assessed patients with HFrEF using the passive leg-lifting maneuver. In this study, paradoxically decreased stroke volume during passive leg lifting was associated with the primary end point of death and HF hospitalization. These studies suggested that the passive leg-lifting maneuver could be used for the risk stratification of patients with HF using E/A (instead of E/e′) and stroke volume (instead of cardiac output). However, the passive leg-lifting maneuver is known to return only up to 200 mL of blood to central circulation.

The author's group developed a novel leg-positive pressure device to continuously increase preload. This device can return more than 500 mL of blood to central circulation, confirmed by simultaneous invasive hemodynamic study. The study showed sufficient ventricular preload led to constant increase in LV end-diastolic pressure in patients with HF.[20,21] After these validation studies, several groups suggested the utility of preload stress echocardiography by leg-positive pressure in HF, VHD, pulmonary hypertension, and so forth.[15,18] For example, in low-flow low-gradient aortic stenosis (AS), dobutamine stress echocardiography is usually used to assess the

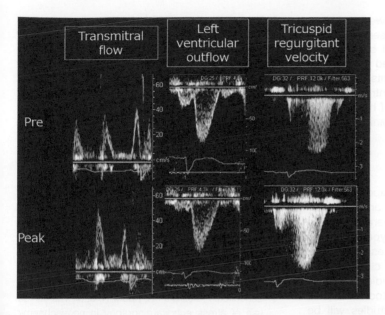

| Transmitral flow | Left ventricular outflow | Tricuspid regurgitant velocity |

Pre

Peak

Fig. 6. A case with leg-positive pressure. The author's group diagnosed severely impaired diastolic dysfunction in the patients using preload stress echocardiography.

true disease severity. Based on the Frank-Starling law, preload stress echocardiography can increase stroke volume and results in an augmentation of mean transvalvular flow rate. Using this increased stroke volume, the projected aortic valve area can be calculated from changes of transvalvular flow rate in AS. The previous report showed the potential usefulness of preload stress echocardiography to distinguish severe or nonsevere AS.[17,40]

A REPRESENTATIVE CASE USING PRELOAD STRESS ECHOCARDIOGRAPHY

A woman in her 70s was referred to the author's hospital with a history of HF (**Fig. 6**). She was free from fatigue in daily activity. LV ejection fraction was preserved. Regional wall motion abnormality was not detected. LV inflow showed E/A was less than 0.8, and E wave was more than 50 cm per second. TR-V was 2.2 m per second. At rest, the author's group diagnosed her with grade I diastolic dysfunction. However, she had repeated HF hospitalizations. The author's group used stress echocardiography in this case. During leg-positive pressure stress, mitral inflow dramatically changed from relaxation abnormality pattern to pseudonormal pattern. E/e' significantly increased from 9 to 15 (estimated PCWP from 13 to 21). LV outflow (cardiac output) gradually decreased and TR-V (sPAP) was increased during the stress. Cardiac output slightly increased from 3.1 L/min to 4.0 L/min. ΔCO/ΔPCWP was 0.1. Based on these results, the author's group diagnosed her with severely impaired diastolic dysfunction.

FUTURE DIRECTIONS

In patients with increased HF risk (eg, LV hypertrophy, diabetes, obesity, and VHD), E/e', TR-V, and stroke volume, observed during stress as markers of diastolic function, may be a useful hint in determining the disease state of HF. To this day, the

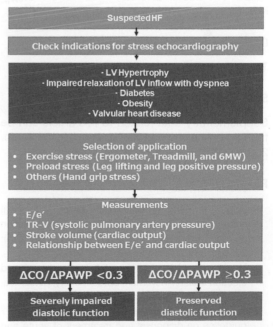

Suspected HF

↓

Check indications for stress echocardiography

↓

· LV Hypertrophy
· Impaired relaxation of LV inflow with dyspnea
· Diabetes
· Obesity
· Valvular heart disease

↓

Selection of application
· Exercise stress (Ergometer, Treadmill, and 6MW)
· Preload stress (Leg lifting and leg positive pressure)
· Others (Hand grip stress)

↓

Measurements
· E/e'
· TR-V (systolic pulmonary artery pressure)
· Stroke volume (cardiac output)
· Relationship between E/e' and cardiac output

| ΔCO/ΔPAWP <0.3 | ΔCO/ΔPAWP ≥0.3 |

| Severely impaired diastolic function | Preserved diastolic function |

Fig. 7. Selection of application for stress echocardiography. The author's group suggest that multipoint assessment of LV filling pressure in relation to cardiac output should be considered for the assessment of heart failure, by using several types of stress application. 6MW, 6-minute walk test.

clinical utility of the relationship between LV filling pressure and cardiac output has been supported by only small and cross-sectional studies. The clinical implications are also limited because of the lack of longitudinal data in patients undergoing medical treatment. Thus, well-controlled multi-center studies with large cohorts of high-risk patients are needed to validate the clinical value of stress echocardiographic data.

SUMMARY

In this comprehensive review, multipoint assessment of LV filling pressure in relation to cardiac output should be taken into consideration for the assessment of HF using several types of stress application (**Fig. 7**). This index makes sense from a physiologic standpoint, and its clinical worth needs to be confirmed in future studies. Exercise echocardiography is an appealing tool for clinical decision making in HF. Further studies will be needed to assess the prognostic value of this method in HF subjects.

ACKNOWLEDGMENTS

The author expresses thanks for the invitation to participate in "Cardiovascular Emergencies Part II" led by Dr Giovanni Esposito and Dr Michinari Hieda. The author acknowledged Robert Zheng, MD, for English editing.

DISCLOSURE

The author has nothing to disclose.

SUPPLEMENTARY DATA

Supplementary data related to this article can be found online at https://doi.org/10.1016/j.hfc.2020.02.001.

REFERENCES

1. Dewan P, Rorth R, Jhund PS, et al. Differential impact of heart failure with reduced ejection fraction on men and women. J Am Coll Cardiol 2019;73(1):29–40.
2. Mentzer G, Hsich EM. Heart failure with reduced ejection fraction in women: epidemiology, outcomes, and treatment. Heart Fail Clin 2019;15(1):19–27.
3. Tsutsui H, Isobe M, Ito H, et al. JCS 2017/JHFS 2017 guideline on diagnosis and treatment of acute and chronic heart failure–digest version. Circ J 2019;83(10):2084–184.
4. Oki T, Miyoshi H, Oishi Y, et al. Heart failure with pre-served ejection fraction—time for a paradigm shift beyond diastolic function. Circ Rep 2019;1(1):8–16.
5. Nagueh SF, Smiseth OA, Appleton CP, et al. Recommendations for the evaluation of left ventricular diastolic function by echocardiography: an update from the American Society of Echocardiography and the European Association of Cardiovascular Imaging. J Am Soc Echocardiogr 2016;29(4):277–314.
6. Bastos MB, Burkhoff D, Maly J, et al. Invasive left ventricle pressure–volume analysis: overview and practical clinical implications. Eur Heart J 2019 Aug 21. pii: ehz552. https://doi.org/10.1093/eurheartj/ehz552.
7. Picano E, Ciampi Q, Citro R, et al. Stress echo 2020: the International Stress Echo Study in ischemic and non-ischemic heart disease. Cardiovasc Ultrasound 2017;15(1):3.
8. Lancellotti P, Dulgheru R, Go YY, et al. Stress echo-cardiography in patients with native valvular heart disease. Heart 2018;104(10):807–13.
9. Lancellotti P, Pellikka PA, Budts W, et al. The clinical use of stress echocardiography in non-ischaemic heart disease: recommendations from the European Association of Cardiovascular Imaging and the American Society of Echocardiography. Eur Heart J Cardiovasc Imaging 2016;17(11):1191–229.
10. Li W, West C, McGhie J, et al. Consensus recommendations for echocardiography in adults with congenital heart defects from the International Society of Adult Congenital Heart Disease (ISACHD). Int J Cardiol 2018;272:77–83.
11. Kusunose K, Yamada H. Rest and exercise echocardiography for early detection of pulmonary hypertension. J Echocardiogr 2016;14(1):2–12.
12. Suzuki T, Izumo M, Suzuki K, et al. Prognostic value of exercise stress echocardiography in patients with secondary mitral regurgitation: a long-term follow-up study. J Echocardiogr 2019;17(3):147–56.
13. Lancellotti P, Pellikka PA, Budts W, et al. The clinical use of stress echocardiography in non-ischaemic heart disease: recommendations from the European Association of Cardiovascular Imaging and the American Society of Echocardiography. J Am Soc Echocardiogr 2017;30(2):101–38.
14. Kelly JP, Andonian BJ, Patel MJ, et al. Trends in cardiorespiratory fitness: the evolution of exercise treadmill testing at a single academic medical center from 1970 to 2012. Am Heart J 2019;210:88–97.
15. Sano H, Tanaka H, Motoji Y, et al. Echocardiography during preload stress for evaluation of right ventricular contractile reserve and exercise capacity in pulmonary hypertension. Echocardiography 2018;35(12):1997–2004.
16. Saijo Y, Yamada H, Kusunose K, et al. A clinical application of preload stress echocardiography for predicting future hemodynamic worsening in patients with early-stage heart failure. Echocardiography 2018;35(10):1587–95.

17. Kusunose K, Yamada H, Nishio S, et al. Preload stress echocardiography predicts outcomes in patients with preserved ejection fraction and low-gradient aortic stenosis. Circ Cardiovasc Imaging 2017;10(10) [pii:e006690].

18. Matsuzoe H, Matsumoto K, Tanaka H, et al. Significant prognostic value of acute preload stress echocardiography using leg-positive pressure maneuver for patients with symptomatic severe aortic stenosis awaiting aortic valve intervention. Circ J 2017; 81(12):1927–35.

19. Henein MY, Tossavainen E, A'Roch R, et al. Can Doppler echocardiography estimate raised pulmonary capillary wedge pressure provoked by passive leg lifting in suspected heart failure? Clin Physiol Funct Imaging 2019;39(2):128–34.

20. Kusunose K, Yamada H, Nishio S, et al. Interval from the onset of transmitral flow to annular velocity is a marker of LV filling pressure. JACC Cardiovasc Imaging 2013;6(4):528–30.

21. Yamada H, Kusunose K, Nishio S, et al. Pre-load stress echocardiography for predicting the prognosis in mild heart failure. JACC Cardiovasc Imaging 2014;7(7):641–9.

22. Penicka M, Bartunek J, Trakalova H, et al. Heart failure with preserved ejection fraction in outpatients with unexplained dyspnea: a pressure-volume loop analysis. J Am Coll Cardiol 2010;55(16):1701–10.

23. Kusunose K, Yamada H, Nishio S, et al. Pulmonary artery hypertension-specific therapy improves exercise tolerance and outcomes in exercise-induced pulmonary hypertension. JACC Cardiovasc Imaging 2019;12(12):2576–9.

24. Keusch S, Bucher A, Müller-Mottet S, et al. Experience with exercise right heart catheterization in the diagnosis of pulmonary hypertension: a retrospective study. Multidiscip Respir Med 2014;9(1):51.

25. Obokata M, Kane GC, Reddy YN, et al. Role of diastolic stress testing in the evaluation for heart failure with preserved ejection fraction: a simultaneous invasive-echocardiographic study. Circulation 2017;135(9):825–38.

26. Eisman AS, Shah RV, Dhakal BP, et al. Pulmonary capillary wedge pressure patterns during exercise predict exercise capacity and incident heart failure. Circ Heart Fail 2018;11(5):e004750.

27. Mullens W, Borowski AG, Curtin RJ, et al. Tissue Doppler imaging in the estimation of intracardiac filling pressure in decompensated patients with advanced systolic heart failure. Circulation 2009; 119(1):62–70.

28. Burgess MI, Jenkins C, Sharman JE, et al. Diastolic stress echocardiography: hemodynamic validation and clinical significance of estimation of ventricular filling pressure with exercise. J Am Coll Cardiol 2006;47(9):1891–900.

29. Nagueh SF, Middleton KJ, Kopelen HA, et al. Doppler tissue imaging: a noninvasive technique for evaluation of left ventricular relaxation and estimation of filling pressures. J Am Coll Cardiol 1997; 30(6):1527–33.

30. Park J-H, Marwick TH. Use and limitations of E/e' to assess left ventricular filling pressure by echocardiography. J Cardiovasc Ultrasound 2011;19(4): 169–73.

31. Erdei T, Smiseth OA, Marino P, et al. A systematic review of diastolic stress tests in heart failure with preserved ejection fraction, with proposals from the EU-FP7 MEDIA study group. Eur J Heart Fail 2014;16(12):1345–61.

32. Gola A, Pozzoli M, Capomolla S, et al. Comparison of Doppler echocardiography with thermodilution for assessing cardiac output in advanced congestive heart failure. Am J Cardiol 1996; 78(6):708–12.

33. Pozzoli M, Capomolla S, Cobelli F, et al. Reproducibility of Doppler indices of left ventricular systolic and diastolic function in patients with severe chronic heart failure. Eur Heart J 1995;16(2):194–200.

34. Bernstein DP. A new stroke volume equation for thoracic electrical bioimpedance: theory and rationale. Crit Care Med 1986;14(10):904–9.

35. Kusunose K, Yamada H, Hotchi J, et al. Prediction of future overt pulmonary hypertension by 6-min walk stress echocardiography in patients with connective tissue disease. J Am Coll Cardiol 2015;66(4): 376–84.

36. Kosmala W, Holland DJ, Rojek A, et al. Effect of If-channel inhibition on hemodynamic status and exercise tolerance in heart failure with preserved ejection fraction: a randomized trial. J Am Coll Cardiol 2013; 62(15):1330–8.

37. Pozzoli M, Capomolla S, Sanarico M, et al. Doppler evaluations of left ventricular diastolic filling and pulmonary wedge pressure provide similar prognostic information in patients with systolic dysfunction after myocardial infarction. Am Heart J 1995;129(4): 716–25.

38. Ishizu T, Seo Y, Kawano S, et al. Stratification of impaired relaxation filling patterns by passive leg lifting in patients with preserved left ventricular ejection fraction. Eur J Heart Fail 2008;10(11):1094–101.

39. Abe Y, Akamatsu K, Furukawa A, et al. Pre-load-induced changes in forward LV stroke and functional mitral regurgitation: echocardiographic detection of the descending limb of Starling's curve. JACC Cardiovasc Imaging 2017;10(6):611–8.

40. Pibarot P, Clavel MA. Preload stress echocardiography: a new tool to confirm severity of low-gradient aortic stenosis. Circ Cardiovasc Imaging 2017; 10(10).

Obesity-Related Heart Failure with Preserved Ejection Fraction
Pathophysiology, Diagnosis, and Potential Therapies

Tomonari Harada, MD, Masaru Obokata, MD, PhD*

KEYWORDS

- Adiposity • Diagnosis • Echocardiography • Inflammation • Natriuretic peptide • Obesity

KEY POINTS

- Obesity and increased adiposity have multiple adverse effects on the cardiovascular system.
- Obesity is increasingly recognized as an important phenotype of heart failure with preserved ejection fraction (HFpEF).
- Many patients with the obesity HFpEF phenotype have normal natriuretic peptide levels, which increases HFpEF diagnostic difficulty.
- Obesity and increased adiposity may be a target for HFpEF, for which there is currently no established treatment.

INTRODUCTION

Heart failure (HF) is a widespread public health problem with increasing burdens of morbidity, mortality, and health care costs. As of 2018, approximately 6.5 million American adults (2.5%) have HF[1]; importantly, its prevalence is expected to continue to increase, affecting more than 8 million people in the United States by 2030.[2] Among HF patients, approximately half have preserved ejection fraction (HFpEF) and its prevalence relative to HF with reduced ejection fraction (HFrEF) is increasing.[3] This epidemic of HFpEF is especially related to the increasing burden of obesity along with population aging and increasing prevalences of other comorbidities such as hypertension, diabetes, and atrial fibrillation.[1,4,5]

Obesity is increasing at an alarming rate in the United States and in most of the Westernized world. Since 1980, the prevalence of obesity has doubled in more than 70 countries; a total of 603.7 million adults (12.0%) were obese in 2015.[5] The United States has the highest proportion of obese adults; currently one-third of American adults are obese (31% of men, 35% of women).[1,5] The prevalence of obesity in patients with HFpEF is estimated to be much higher (~50%).[6] Obesity and increased adiposity adversely affect the cardiovascular system and can contribute to the pathophysiology of HFpEF, making obesity-related HFpEF a distinct phenotype in this substantially heterogeneous syndrome.[7] Considering its high prevalence and pathophysiologic significance, it is increasingly recognized that obesity

Department of Cardiovascular Medicine, Gunma University, Graduate School of Medicine, 3-39-22 Showa-Machi, Maebashi, Gunma 371-8511, Japan
* Corresponding author.
E-mail address: obokata.masaru@gunma-u.ac.jp

Heart Failure Clin 16 (2020) 357–368
https://doi.org/10.1016/j.hfc.2020.02.004
1551-7136/20/© 2020 Elsevier Inc. All rights reserved.

and increased adiposity may be a key therapeutic target for patients with HFpEF.[8,9]

Unlike HFrEF, making the diagnosis of HFpEF, especially in patients without overt congestion, is difficult.[10–12] The presence of obesity complicates the interpretation of natriuretic peptide levels and echocardiographic parameters; thus, making the diagnosis of obesity-related HFpEF becomes more challenging.[7,13] For these reasons, this review focuses on obesity-related HFpEF and describes the impacts of obesity and adiposity on the pathophysiology of HFpEF. The authors also discuss diagnosis of HFpEF as well as potential treatments for the HFpEF-obesity phenotype.

Pathophysiology of Obesity-Related Heart Failure with Preserved Ejection Fraction: Hemodynamic Effects

Obesity and excessive fat accumulation can contribute to the pathophysiology of HFpEF through hemodynamic, inflammatory, mechanical, and neurohormonal effects (**Fig. 1**). Plasma volume expansion may be a primary driver of hemodynamic alterations that predispose affected individuals to obesity-related changes in cardiac structure and function. Plasma volume expansion in patients with obesity-related HFpEF can lead to chamber remodeling.[7] Left ventricular (LV) hypertrophy in these patients can be concentric[14–16] or eccentric,[17] but visceral adiposity is likely to be more associated with concentric remodeling.[18] Importantly, increased LV mass is associated with adverse outcomes in HFpEF regardless of hypertrophy type.[19,20] Plasma volume expansion in obesity-related HFpEF may also adversely affect LV diastolic function. It is noteworthy that body fat distribution is a key factor in obesity-related metabolic and cardiovascular diseases and that the effects of obesity on diastolic dysfunction are even more pronounced with increases in central or visceral adiposity.[21–23] Recent data have demonstrated associations between body mass index (BMI) and right ventricular (RV) systolic dysfunction and dilation in HFpEF.[7,24] This may support a role of increased plasma volume driving the obesity-related RV dysfunction. RV dilation, LV dilation, and hypertrophy can lead to enhanced pericardial restraint and diastolic ventricular interdependence by increasing total heart volume, contributing to further elevations in LV filling pressure in obesity-related HFpEF.[7,25] Volume overload also directly causes cardiopulmonary congestion that results in acute decompensation requiring HF hospitalizations.[26]

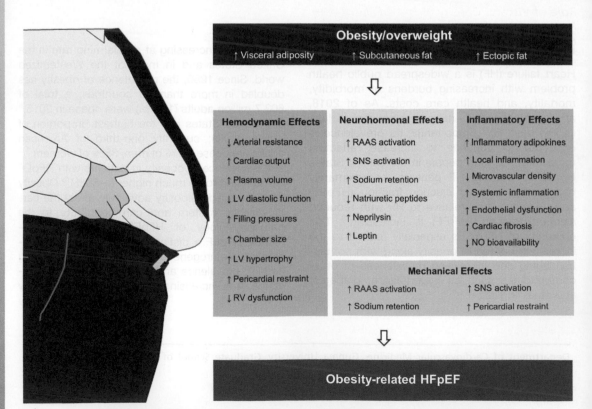

Fig. 1. Adverse effects of obesity and increased adiposity on the cardiovascular system in HFpEF.

The increase in circulating plasma volume in obese patients with HFpEF is likely to be driven by sodium retention and systemic vasodilation.[7,27–29] Excessive systemic vasodilation occurs to meet increased metabolic demands and higher tissue oxygen consumption in obese subjects, which then increases cardiac output.[7,30] Perivascular adipose tissues are known to release several adipokines that induce vasodilation.[31,32] Obesity, especially when associated with intraabdominal fat, contributes to neurohormonal activation, which includes increased sympathetic nervous system (SNS) activity, renin-angiotensin-aldosterone system (RAAS) activation, and an increased synthesis of adipokines that activate the former 2 systems (eg, leptin, aldosterone).[29,33] These alterations in addition to other mechanisms, such as renal compression by the accumulation of perirenal, visceral, and retroperitoneal fat and degradation of endogenous natriuretic peptides by adipocyte-derived neprilysin, promote renal sodium reabsorption and result in plasma volume expansion.[29,34–36] Increased sodium reabsorption along with SNS activation can also lead to blood shift from the splanchnic vascular compartment to the central circulation and predispose HF exacerbations.[26]

Role of Visceral Obesity in Heart Failure with Preserved Ejection Fraction: Inflammatory Effects

In the current HFpEF paradigm, obesity is considered a primary driver of the pathophysiology of HFpEF through its inflammatory effect.[37] Systemic inflammation and subsequent coronary microvascular inflammation and dysfunction may promote alterations in cardiomyocyte signaling pathways and myocardium inflammation and fibrosis, leading to myocardial dysfunction and remodeling as well as systemic endothelial dysfunction.[38–41] In particular, an increased visceral adiposity is associated with adipose tissue dysfunction, promoting the upregulation of proinflammatory adipokines (eg, leptin, tumor necrosis factor-α [TNF-α], interleukin-6 [IL-6], and resistin) and the downregulation of antiinflammatory adipokines (eg, adiponectin, omentin-1), leading to a chronic low-grade systemic inflammation.[42] Indeed, it has been shown that visceral fat is larger in obesity-related HFpEF patients than in obese subjects without HF and that proinflammatory markers are further elevated in obese versus nonobese HFpEF patients.[43,44] More importantly, increasing visceral adipose tissue measured by computed tomography was associated with incident HFpEF among the general population, and the presence

of abdominal obesity was associated with increased mortality in established HFpEF.[45,46] In contrast, weight reduction via caloric restriction or aerobic exercise reduced inflammatory markers, improved exercise capacity, and enhanced quality of life in patients with obese HFpEF.[47] Collectively, these findings support the importance of visceral adiposity in the pathophysiology of HFpEF, especially in patients with the HFpEF obesity phenotype.

Further support of the adverse effects of visceral adiposity on HFpEF pathophysiology comes from serial observational studies in Asian HFpEF populations.[48–50] In striking contrast to Western HFpEF populations, most Asian HFpEF patients have a normal body weight. In a recent multinational registry of Asian HF patients (ASIAN-HF registry), the prevalence of obesity (BMI >30 kg/m^2) was extremely low in Asian HFpEF populations, especially those in Southeast Asia (16.5% Japan/Korea).[48] It has been consistently reported that Asians have larger abdominal and visceral fat volumes and worse insulin resistance than Westerners of similar BMI.[51–53] This may explain the much higher rates of type 2 diabetes in an Asian HFpEF population than a Caucasian population (62% vs 26%) despite the lower prevalence of obesity.[49] The multinational registry has shown the so-called obesity paradox in which a higher BMI is associated with reduced cardiovascular events.[50] However, it also demonstrated that cardiovascular events increase with increasing waist-to-height ratio,[50] which supports the concept that the relatively large amount of visceral adiposity and its metabolic and inflammatory consequences, rather than BMI alone, are central players to the pathophysiology of Asian HFpEF patients. Further studies are required to understand the importance of visceral adiposity, especially in Asian HFpEF patients, by directly comparing the amount of visceral adiposity and its adverse effect on cardiac structure, function, and hemodynamics between Asian and Western HFpEF populations.

In addition to systemic inflammation, the accumulation of ectopic fat is another important characteristic in obesity, and epicardial fat in particular is an emerging area of investigation in obesity-related HFpEF.[54] Epicardial adipose tissue promotes the upregulation of proinflammatory cytokines such as IL-1β, IL-6, and TNF-α.[55,56] The lack of fascia between the epicardial fat and the myocardium or adventitia may allow direct diffusion of proinflammatoryadipokines into the adjacent myocardium or coronary microcirculation in a paracrine-like manner.[57,58] Epicardial fat deposits are closely associated with cardiac inflammation in obese mice model and cardiac fibrosis in patients with chronic HF.[56,59] A recent study demonstrated a larger epicardial adipose tissue volume in HFpEF versus metabolic syndrome patients without HF and reported that a greater volume of epicardial adipose tissue is correlated with worse myocardial function assessed by speckle tracking echocardiography.[60] In addition to the inflammatory effects, epicardial fat accumulation may have deleterious mechanical effects as a space-occupying lesion.[7] Increased epicardial fat along with cardiomegaly in obese patients with HFpEF was shown to cause space limitations in the pericardial sac and lead to pericardial restraint and enhanced diastolic ventricular interdependence.[7] Importantly, the enhanced pericardial restraint may worsen during exercise, which further increases LV filling pressure with exercise. Obesity and increased adiposity are also associated with increased inflammation within the skeletal muscle,[38,61–63] and the importance of skeletal muscle inflammation in HFpEF was reviewed in detail elsewhere.[64]

Neurohormonal Effects

Increased neurohormonal activation may play an important role in obese HFpEF.[65] Several mediators have been suggested, including SNS activation, RAAS activation, and an increased release of adipokines such as leptin, TNF-α, and IL-6.[29,66] Neurohormonal activation may contribute to the cardiac structural remodeling observed in obese patients with HFpEF by inducing cardiac fibrosis, sodium retention–mediated plasma volume expansion, and systemic hypertension. Studies have shown that leptin is an important player of neurohormonal activation, whereas hyperleptinemia contributes to obesity-related cardiovascular disease in which leptin enhances both RAAS and renal SNS and promotes cardiomyocyte hypertrophy and fibrosis.[67–70] Interestingly, leptin levels are reportedly elevated in patients with HFpEF.[71] Despite the expectation of adverse effects of neurohormonal activation in obesity-related HFpEF, extensive data exist in obesity in general, and previous studies directly comparing these factors between obese and nonobese HFpEF patients are limited.[44] Indeed, obese HFpEF patients did not display greater neurohormonal activation than nonobese HFpEF, demonstrating similar plasma levels of endothelin and aldosterone.[44]

Neprilysin is responsible for the degradation and inactivation of many bioactive peptides, including endothelin, angiotensins, and natriuretic peptides. The inhibition of neprilysin increases diuresis, vasodilation, and natriuresis by enhancing biologically active natriuretic peptides, which may reduce HF hospitalizations in patients with HFpEF.[72,73] Plasma and adipose tissue neprilysin levels are reported to be increased with increasing BMI.[35] As such, obese HFpEF patients were more likely to benefit from neprilysin inhibition if they had higher baseline levels. Because the presence of obesity and BMI were not included in prespecified subgroup analyses in the PARAGON-HF trial,[73] further post-hoc analyses may be of interest.

Diagnostic Challenge in Obese Patients with Heart Failure with Preserved Ejection Fraction

The diagnosis of HFpEF is obvious in patients with overt congestion in whom jugular vein distention, peripheral edema, and pulmonary edema are present at rest. In contrast, the identification of HFpEF among euvolemic patients with exertional dyspnea remains challenging.[12,74] This diagnostic difficulty in HFpEF is related to the fact that shortness of breath, a primary symptom of HF, is not specific to HFpEF; there are various differential diagnoses among patients with normal EF, and LV filling pressures are often normal at rest but become increased only during the stress of exercise.[10] The presence of obesity further complicates diagnosis of HFpEF. This is because physical examination as well as electrocardiogram, chest radiograph, and echocardiographic findings may be less reliable in obese patients,[75,76] and the interpretations of natriuretic peptide levels and echocardiographic findings can be complicated.[7,44] Although exertional dyspnea is a common symptom among obese patients,[77] approximately half of HFpEF patients are obese; more importantly, the presence of obesity in dyspneic patients increases their probability of having HFpEF.[12] Therefore, special attention should be paid to patients presenting with dyspnea and obesity, as it is important to identify HFpEF among them. In the diagnostic evaluation, care should be taken to exclude other differential diagnoses (**Table 1**). In addition to HF, it is important to remember that obesity is a risk factor for other cardiovascular diseases that mimic HFpEF, such as coronary artery disease, pulmonary embolism, and aortic stenosis.[78]

Natriuretic Peptide Levels in the Evaluation of Obesity-Related Heart Failure with Preserved Ejection Fraction

The natriuretic peptide level is often used as an initial test in the diagnosis of HFpEF. The European Society of Cardiology (ESC) guidelines propose that natriuretic peptide level can be used to exclude HFpEF because of its very high negative

Table 1
Differential diagnoses of obese heart failure with preserved ejection fraction and key testings considered

Differential Diagnosis	Association with Obesity	Key Testings Considered
High-output heart failure	++	Natriuretic peptides, TTE, RHC
Valvular heart disease[a]	++	TTE, TEE
Coronary artery disease	+	TTE, coronary angiography
Constrictive pericarditis	+	TTE, RHC
Pulmonary thromboembolism	+	CT, TTE
Pulmonary arterial hypertension	+	TTE, RHC, CT
Chronic thromboembolic pulmonary hypertension	?[b]	V/Q scan, high-resolution CT, RHC ± pulmonary angiography
Chronic obstructive pulmonary disease	+	Spirometry, high-resolution CT

Abbreviations: CT, computed tomography; RHC, right heart catheterization; TEE, transesophageal echocardiography; TTE, transthoracic echocardiography; V/Q scan, ventilation/perfusion scintigraphy.

[a] Obesity is reported to be a strong risk factor of especially aortic stenosis.

[b] Although obesity is strongly associated with deep vein thrombosis (DVT) and DVT is a primary risk factor of chronic thromboembolic pulmonary hypertension (CTEPH), data supporting a direct cause-effect relationship between obesity and CTEPH are scarce.

Data from Larsson SC, Burgess S, Ba M, Rees JMB, Mason AM. Body mass index and body composition in relation to 14 CV conditions in UK Biobank. Eur. Heart J. 2020;41:221–6.

predictive value.[79] However, it is noteworthy that most studies supporting this notion included HFrEF and focused on identifying systolic dysfunction rather than HFpEF.[80–82] A robust body of data repeatedly demonstrated that many patients with compensated or even decompensated HFpEF have normal natriuretic peptide levels.[10,13,74] Furthermore, obese patients have lower natriuretic peptide levels than their nonobese counterparts regardless of HF status,[83–85] and natriuretic peptide concentration is reportedly much lower in obese HFpEF patients than in nonobese HFpEF patients.[7] This may be explained by enhanced natriuretic peptide degradation in the adipose tissue, suppression of natriuretic peptide generation by androgen, insulin resistance or hyperinsulinism, or lower myocardial wall stress from pericardial restraint and heightened pericardial restraint.[7,86,87] Collectively, the consensus that natriuretic peptide concentration is useful as a rule-out test is not consistent with empirical data, which may lead to a serious underdiagnosis of HFpEF.

Clinically, care should be taken in cases of lower natriuretic peptide concentrations in dyspnea patients with a BMI greater than or equal to 30 kg/m^2. A recent recommendation from the Heart Failure Association of the ESC suggested the use of lower cut-off concentrations in obese patients (about 50% lower) to optimize sensitivity, although this change compromises specificity.[88] Notably, compared with nonobese patients with HFpEF,

obese patients with HFpEF displayed higher LV filling pressure at any natriuretic peptide value.[7] This may lead to a higher incidence of worse outcomes at a given level of natriuretic peptide in obese HFpEF patients than in their nonobese counterparts.[89]

Other Potential Biomarkers for the Diagnosis of Obesity-Related Heart Failure with Preserved Ejection Fraction

Other candidate biomarkers that may be useful for identifying HFpEF among dyspneic patients with obesity include midregional proatrial natriuretic peptide (MR-proANP) and growth differentiation factor 15 (GDF-15). The Biomarkers in Acute Congestive Heart Failure trial demonstrated that MR-proANP had additive value for diagnosing acute HF when used with brain natriuretic peptide (BNP) values in 1641 obese dyspneic patients.[90] In the ProBNP Investigation of Acute Dyspnoea in the Emergency Department trial, however, the sensitivity of MR-proANP for diagnosing acute HF was reduced in patients with a BMI greater than or equal to 30 kg/m^2 compared with the overall cohort (73% vs 82%, respectively), although its diagnostic accuracy remained good (C-statistic, 0.90).[91] On the other hand, the Obesity Weight Reduction and Remodeling Study, which included obese patients with a mean BMI of 40.3 kg/m^2, reported that GDF-15 had a superior diagnostic ability to identify possible HFpEF cases compared with NT-proBNP (area under the curve, 0.698 vs 0.562).[92] Furthermore, the addition of GDF-15 to clinically established risk factors (age, sex, BMI, type 2 diabetes, and systolic blood pressure) improved its discriminative ability among obese patients. Further studies are needed to establish biomarkers for identifying HFpEF among obese dyspneic patients.

Echocardiography in the Diagnostic Evaluation of Obese Heart Failure with Preserved Ejection Fraction

Echocardiography provides information about cardiac structure and function and plays a fundamental role in the diagnostic evaluation of HFpEF.[93] It is possible that diagnostic-quality images cannot be obtained in a proportion of obese patients even when performed by well-trained sonographers. Even when feasibly obtained, echocardiographic indices could be less reliable. Recent data raised serious questions regarding accuracy of the contemporary echocardiographic standards for the diagnosis of HFpEF. In recent studies validating the diagnostic accuracy of the guidelines against the gold standard of invasively measured filling pressure, although specificity was high, sensitivity was consistently low (10%–57% for the American Society of Echocardiography/European Association of Cardiovascular Imaging).[74,94–96] The fact that many patients with HFpEF have normal filling pressure at rest can explain the lower sensitivity,[74] but LA volume index may be a major contributor to the poor sensitivity by seriously underestimating true LA size in obese patients with a larger body surface area.[95] In fact, an ancillary study of the Phosphodiesterase-5 Inhibition to Improve Clinical Status and Exercise Capacity in Heart Failure with Preserved Ejection Fraction (RELAX) trial demonstrated a much smaller LA volume index in obese patients with HFpEF than in their nonobese counterparts (38 mL/m² vs 54 mL/m², $P<.001$) despite more severe signs and symptoms of HF as well as reduced exercise capacity (lower peak oxygen consumption and shorter 6-minute walk distance).[44] Further studies are required to determine the reasonable indexations of LA volume such as for height among patients with HFpEF.[97]

Lung ultrasound as a potential tool to identify heart failure with preserved ejection fraction among obese patients

Accumulating evidence has shown that increases in interstitial lung water at rest or even during exercise can be reliably detected by lung ultrasound as multiple B-lines in patients with HF.[98] A previous meta-analysis examining 1914 dyspneic patients referred to the emergency department demonstrated that the B-line profile is the top useful modality to identify cardiogenic origin dyspnea, boasting 85% sensitivity and 92% specificity.[99] In recent studies using the gold standard of invasively measured LV filling pressure, increases in B-lines were associated with higher LV filling pressure at rest and during exercise in obese patients with HFpEF (mean BMI, 31–35 kg/m²).[100,101] This finding suggests that lung ultrasound may be less influenced by patient's body habitus and thus can be a useful modality in diagnostic evaluations among obese patients.[98] It is important to remember that multiple B-lines reflect a consequence of interstitial syndrome (cardiogenic pulmonary edema, acute respiratory distress syndrome, or pneumonia) rather than a disease; thus, clinicians must differentiate among these conditions.[98] Increases in pulmonary edema are also associated with reduced cardiac output reserve, worse exercise capacity, and adverse outcomes in HFpEF patients[100,102] and are currently being evaluated as a surrogate marker to guide intervention or even serve as a novel treatment target.

Potential Treatments for Obesity-Related Heart Failure with Preserved Ejection Fraction

It is increasingly recognized that HFpEF is a heterogeneous syndrome, and subgrouping patients into pathophysiologically homogeneous groups may be a promising approach to maximize the therapeutic benefits in people with HFpEF, for which there is no established treatment to improve prognosis.[8] Considering its high prevalence and pathophysiologic significance as described earlier, obesity is now appreciated as an important clinical phenotype of HFpEF and can be a key target for therapy. There are several possible treatments targeting obesity-related HFpEF (**Table 2**). Intentional weight loss achieved by caloric restriction or exercise has been shown to improve exercise capacity and quality of life in obesity-related HFpEF.[47] Bariatric surgery might hold promise in terms of its substantial weight reduction and sustained effect.[103] Other potential therapies include diuretics or sodium-glucose cotransporter-2 inhibitors for hypervolemic state, antiinflammatory drugs such as statins for systemic inflammation, and neurohormonal antagonists such as neprilysin inhibitors.[37,65,72,104–106]

However, controversy persists regarding the existence of the obesity paradox, in which some studies have demonstrated that mild obesity is paradoxically associated with decreased mortality compared with normal weight in HFpEF.[6,107] As

Table 2
Potential therapies for obesity-related HFpEF

Intervention	Expected Therapeutic Effects
Exercise and/or diet	↓Body weight, ↑Exercise capacity, ↑Quality of life
Bariatric surgery	↓↓Body weight
Diuretics	↓Plasma volume
SGLT-2 inhibitors	↓Plasma volume, ↓Body weight, ↓Visceral adiposity, ↑Renal function ↓Systemic inflammation
Statins	↓Systemic inflammation
Neprilysin inhibitors	↓Plasma volume
Mineralocorticoid receptor antagonists	↓Plasma volume, ↓Sodium retention, ↓Systemic inflammation

Abbreviations: SGLT-2, sodium-glucose transporter-2: and other abbreviations as in **Table 1**.

Table 3
Key questions and knowledge gaps with regard to the diagnosis of HFpEF

Key Questions	Knowledge Gaps and Future Studies Needed
Obese HFpEF patients can have normal natriuretic peptide levels. What is the most practical way not to miss the presence of HFpEF?	In obese patients who have signs and symptoms of HF with normal natriuretic peptides, clinicians must remain vigilant and use echocardiography and/or invasive hemodynamic testing to assess objective evidence of elevated LV filling pressures.
Are there optimal cutoff values for natriuretic peptides to diagnose HFpEF among obese patients?	There is no established cutoff for natriuretic peptides specific to obese patients. A recent recommendation suggests the use of lower cut-off concentrations (about 50% lower) to optimize sensitivity.
Are there biomarkers that may help to diagnose obese HFpEF?	MR-proANP and GDF-15 can be potential biomarkers for identifying HFpEF among obese patients. Further studies are needed to search novel biomarkers to diagnose HFpEF.
Diagnostic-quality echocardiographic images could not be obtained and echocardiographic indices could be less reliable in a proportion of obese patients. What are the roles of different modalities in the evaluation for obese HFpEF?	Other imaging modalities such as cardiac magnetic resonance, cardiac computed tomography, and positron emission tomography may be promising, but the data to support their usefulness require further investigation.
Why is LA volume index less sensitive for the diagnosis of HFpEF among obese patients?	Indexations of LA volume can lead to a serious underestimation of true LA size in obese patients with a larger body surface area. Further studies are required to determine the reasonable indexations of LA volume among patients with HFpEF.
Are there echocardiographic techniques that may help to diagnose obese HFpEF?	Echocardiographic B-lines by lung ultrasound may be promising, but further research is needed to establish the roles of lung ultrasound in the HFpEF diagnostic approach.

Abbreviations: GDF-15, growth differentiation factor-15; LA, left atrial; MR-proANP, mid-regional pro-atrial natriuretic peptide; and other abbreviations as in **Table 1**.

such, some investigators have suggested caution in aggressively treating excess adiposity in patients with HFpEF.[108] However, the association between BMI and mortality in HFpEF was U-shaped,[6,109] and there was a linear relationship between abdominal obesity and outcome in HFpEF,[46,50] which suggests that abdominal obesity and at least morbid obesity may be a target for therapy in HFpEF. Further studies are required to improve outcomes in this population.

SUMMARY

The prevalence of both obesity and HFpEF is growing at an alarming pace worldwide, and most current patients with HFpEF are obese. Historically, obesity has been considered merely a common comorbidity for HFpEF rather than a cause of cardiovascular derangement. However, it is now recognized that obesity is the most common and clinically important phenotype of HFpEF and that it has distinct pathophysiological mechanisms as described in this article. The diagnosis of HFpEF is challenging, especially among obese dyspneic patients. There are many key questions and knowledge gaps in evidence with regard to the diagnosis of obesity-related HFpEF, and further studies are needed to answer these questions (**Table 3**). Finally, therapies targeting overall adiposity or obesity-driven adverse effects may be promising for this growing phenotype.

ACKNOWLEDGMENTS

Dr M. Obokata has received research grants from Fukuda Foundation for Medical Technology and Mochida Memorial Foundation for Medical and Pharmaceutical Research.

DISCLOSURE

The authors have nothing to disclose.

REFERENCES

1. Benjamin EJ, Virani SS, Callaway CW, et al. Heart disease and stroke statistics - 2018 update: a report from the American Heart Association. Circulation 2018;137(12):e67–492.

2. Bluemke DA, Butler J, Frcp C, et al. Forecasting the impact of heart failure in the United States: a policy statement from the American Heart Association. Circ Heart Fail 2014;6:606–19.

3. Steinberg BA, Zhao X, Heidenreich PA, et al. Trends in patients hospitalized with heart failure and preserved left ventricular ejection fraction: prevalence, therapies, and outcomes. Circulation 2012;126:65–75.

4. Dunlay SM, Roger VL, Redfield MM. Epidemiology of heart failure with preserved ejection fraction. Nat Rev Cardiol 2017;14:591–602.

5. Article O. Health effects of overweight and obesity in 195 countries over 25 years. N Engl J Med 2017; 377:13–27.

6. Haass M, Kitzman DW, Anand IS, et al. Body mass index and adverse cardiovascular outcomes in heart failure patients with preserved ejection fraction results from the irbesartan in heart failure with preserved ejection fraction (I-PRESERVE) trial. Circ Heart Fail 2011;4:324–31.

7. Obokata M, Reddy YNV, Pislaru SV, et al. Evidence supporting the existence of a distinct obese phenotype of heart failure with preserved ejection fraction. Circulation 2017;136:6–19.

8. Shah SJ, Kitzman DW, Borlaug BA, et al. Phenotype-specific treatment of heart failure with preserved ejection fraction. Circulation 2016;134: 73–90.

9. Obokata M, Reddy YNV, Borlaug BA. Diastolic dysfunction and heart failure with preserved ejection fraction. JACCCardiovascImaging 2020;13: 245–57.

10. Borlaug BA, Nishimura RA, Sorajja P, et al. Exercise hemodynamics enhance diagnosis of early heart failure with preserved ejection fraction. Circ Heart Fail 2010;3:588–95.

11. Obokata M, Reddy YNV, Borlaug BA. The role of echocardiography in heart failure with preserved ejection fraction: what do we want from imaging? Heart Fail Clin 2019;15:241–56.

12. Reddy YNV, Carter RE, Obokata M, et al. A simple, evidence-based approach to help guide diagnosis of heart failure with preserved ejection fraction. Circulation 2018;138:861–70.

13. Anjan VY, Loftus TM, Burke MA, et al. Prevalence, clinical phenotype, and outcomes associated with normal B-type natriuretic peptide levels in heart failure with preserved ejection fraction. Am J Cardiol 2012;110:870–6.

14. Turkbey EB, McClelland RL, Kronmal RA, et al. The impact of obesity on the left ventricle.the multiethnic study of atherosclerosis (MESA). JACCCardiovascImaging 2010;3:266–74.

15. Peterson LR, Waggoner AD, Schechtman KB, et al. Alterations in left ventricular structure and function in young healthy obese women: Assessment by echocardiography and tissue Doppler imaging. J Am CollCardiol 2004;43:1399–404.

16. Wong CY, O'Moore-Sullivan T, Leano R, et al. Alterations of left ventricular myocardial characteristics associated with obesity. Circulation 2004;110: 3081–7.

17. Duflou J, Virmani R, Rabin I, et al. Sudden death as a result of heart disease in morbid obesity. Am Heart J 1995;130:306–13.

18. Neeland IJ, Gupta S, Ayers CR, et al. Relation of regional fat distribution to left ventricular structure and function. CircCardiovascImaging 2013;6:800–7.

19. Zile MR, Gottdiener JS, Hetzel SJ, et al. Prevalence and significance of alterations in cardiac structure and function in patients with heart failure and a preserved ejection fraction. Circulation 2011;124: 2491–501.

20. Shah AM, Claggett B, Sweitzer NK, et al. Prognostic importance of impaired systolic function in heart failure with preserved ejection fraction and the impact of spironolactone. Circulation 2015; 132:402–14.

21. Wohlfahrt P, Redfield MM, Lopez-Jimenez F, et al. Impact of general and central adiposity onventricular-arterial aging in women and men. JACC Heart Fail 2014;2:490–9.

22. Morricone L, Malavazos AE, Coman C, et al. Echocardiographic abnormalities in normotensive obese patients: relationship with visceral fat. Obes Res 2002;10:489–98.

23. Selvaraj S, Martinez EE, Aguilar FG, et al. Association of central adiposity with adverse cardiac mechanics: findings from the HyperGEN Study. CircCardiovascImaging 2016;9 [pii:e004396].

24. Gorter TM, Hoendermis ES, van Veldhuisen DJ, et al. Right ventricular dysfunction in heart failure with preserved ejection fraction: a systematic review and meta-analysis. Eur J Heart Fail 2016;18: 1472–87.

25. Melenovsky V, Borlaug BA, Rosen B, et al. Cardiovascular features of heart failure with preserved ejection fraction versus nonfailing hypertensive left ventricular hypertrophy in the urban baltimore community. the role of atrial remodeling/dysfunction. J Am CollCardiol 2007;49:198–207.

26. Fudim M, Hernandez AF, Felker GM. Role of volume redistribution in the congestion of heart failure. J Am HeartAssoc 2017;6:e006817.

27. Licata G, Scaglione R, Barbagallo M, et al. Effect of obesity on left ventricular function studied by radionuclide angiocardiography. Int J Obes 1991;15: 295–302.

28. Maurer MS, King DL, El-KhouryRumbarger L, et al. Left heart failure with a normal ejection fraction: Identification of different pathophysiologic mechanisms. J Card Fail 2005;11:177–87.

29. Hall JE, Do Carmo JM, Da Silva AA, et al. Obesity-induced hypertension: interaction of neurohumoral and renal mechanisms. Circ Res 2015;116: 991–1006.

30. Reddy YNV, Melenovsky V, Redfield MM, et al. High-output heart failure: a 15-year experience. J Am CollCardiol 2016;68:473–82.

31. Lembo G, Vecchione C, Fratta L, et al. Leptin induces direct vasodilation through distinct endothelial mechanisms. Diabetes 2000;49:293–7.

32. Gollasch M. Vasodilator signals from perivascular adipose tissue. Br J Pharmacol 2012;165:633–42.

33. Xie D, Bollag WB. Obesity, hypertension and aldosterone: Is leptin the link? J Endocrinol 2016;230: F7–11.

34. Chandra A, Neeland IJ, Berry JD, et al. The relationship of body mass and fat distribution with incident hypertension: Observations from the dallas heart study. J Am CollCardiol 2014;64:997–1002.

35. Standeven KF, Hess K, Carter AM, et al. Neprilysin, obesity and the metabolic syndrome. Int J Obes 2011;35:1031–40.

36. Foster MC, Hwang SJ, Porter SA, et al. Fatty kidney, hypertension, and chronic kidney disease: the framingham heart study. Hypertension 2011; 58:784–90.

37. Paulus WJ, Tschöpe C. A novel paradigm for heart failure with preserved ejection fraction: comorbidities drive myocardial dysfunction and remodeling through coronary microvascular endothelial inflammation. J Am CollCardiol 2013;62:263–71.

38. Kitzman DW, Nicklas B, Kraus WE, et al. Skeletal muscle abnormalities and exercise intolerance in older patients with heart failure and preserved ejection fraction. Am JPhysiol HeartCircPhysiol 2014;306:H1364–70.

39. Virdis A, Duranti E, Rossi C, et al. Tumour necrosis factor-alpha participates on the endothelin-1/nitric oxide imbalance in small arteries from obese patients: Role of perivascular adipose tissue. EurHeart J 2015;36:784–94.

40. Van Dijk CGM, Oosterhuis NR, Xu YJ, et al. Distinct endothelial cell responses in the heart and kidney microvasculature characterize the progression of heart failure with preserved ejection fraction in the obese ZSF1 rat with cardiorenal metabolic syndrome. Circ Heart Fail 2016;9:1–13.

41. Badimon L, Bugiardini R, Cenko E, et al. Position paper of the European Society of Cardiology-working group of coronary pathophysiology and microcirculation: obesity and heart disease. EurHeart J 2017;38:1951–1958a.

42. Ouchi N, Parker JL, Lugus JJ, et al. Adipokines in inflammation and metabolic disease. Nat Rev Immunol 2011;11:85–97.

43. Haykowsky MJ, Nicklas BJ, Brubaker PH, et al. Regional adipose distribution and its relationship to exercise intolerance in older obese patients who have heart failure with preserved ejection fraction. JACC Heart Fail 2018;001420:1–10.

44. Reddy YNV, Lewis GD, Shah SJ, et al. Characterization of the obese phenotype of heart failure with preserved ejection fraction: a RELAX Trial Ancillary Study. MayoClinProc 2019;94:1199–209.

45. Rao VN, Zhao D, Allison MA, et al. Adiposity and incident heart failure and its subtypes. JACC Heart Fail 2018;6:942.

46. Tsujimoto T, Kajio H. Abdominal obesity is associated with an increased risk of all-cause mortality in patients with HFpEF. J Am CollCardiol 2017;70:2739–49.

47. Kitzman DW, Brubaker P, Morgan T, et al. Effect of caloric restriction or aerobic exercise training on peak oxygen consumption and quality of life in obese older patients with heart failure with preserved ejection fraction: a randomized clinical trial. JAMA 2016;315:36–46.

48. Tromp J. Heart failure with preserved ejection fraction in Asia. Heart Fail Clin 2019;15:9–18.

49. Bank IEM, Gijsberts CM, Teng THK, et al. Prevalence and clinical significance of diabetes in asian versus white patients with heart failure. JACC Heart Fail 2017;5:14–24.

50. Chandramouli C, Tay WT, Bamadhaj NS, et al. Association of obesity with heart failure outcomes in 11 Asian regions: A cohort study. PLoS Med 2019;16(9):e1002916.

51. Tanaka S, Horimai C, Katsukawa F. Ethnic differences in abdominal visceral fat accumulation between Japanese, African-Americans, and Caucasians: a meta-analysis. ActaDiabetol 2003;40(Suppl 1):S302–4.

52. Kadowaki T, Sekikawa A, Murata K, et al. Japanese men have larger areas of visceral adipose tissue than Caucasian men in the same levels of waist circumference in a population-based study. Int J Obes 2006;30:1163–5.

53. Kadowaki S, Miura K, Kadowaki T, et al. International comparison of abdominal fat distribution among four populations: the ERA-JUMP Study. MetabSyndrRelatDisord 2018;16:166–73.

54. Packer M. Epicardialadipose tissue may mediate deleterious effects of obesity and inflammation on the myocardium. J Am CollCardiol 2018;71:2360–72.

55. Mazurek T, Zhang LF, Zalewski A, et al. Human epicardial adipose tissue is a source of inflammatory mediators. Circulation 2003;108:2460–6.

56. Patel VB, Mori J, McLean BA, et al. ACE2 deficiency worsens epicardial adipose tissue inflammation and cardiac dysfunction in response to diet-induced obesity. Diabetes 2016;65:85–95.

57. Venteclef N, Guglielmi V, Balse E, et al. Human epicardial adipose tissue induces fibrosis of the atrial myocardium through the secretion of adipo-fibrokines. EurHeart J 2015;36:795–805.

58. Iacobellis G. Local and systemic effects of the multifaceted epicardial adipose tissue depot. Nat Rev Endocrinol 2015;11:363–71.

59. Wu CK, Tsai HY, Su MYM, et al. Evolutional change in epicardial fat and its correlation with myocardial diffuse fibrosis in heart failure patients. J ClinLipidol 2017;11:1421–31.

60. Hung CL, Yun CH, Lai YH, et al. An observational study of the association among interatrial adiposity by computed tomography measure, insulin resistance, and left atrial electromechanical disturbances in heart failure. Medicine(Baltimore) 2016;95:1–11.

61. Wu H, Ballantyne CM. Skeletal muscle inflammation and insulin resistance in obesity. J Clin Invest 2017;127:43–54.

62. Haykowsky MJ, Brubaker PH, Stewart KP, et al. Effect of endurance training on the determinants of peak exercise oxygen consumption in elderly patients with stable compensated heart failure and preserved ejection fraction. J Am CollCardiol 2012;60:120–8.

63. Haykowsky MJ, Kouba EJ, Brubaker PH, et al. Skeletal muscle composition and its relation to exercise intolerance in older patients with heart failure and preserved ejection fraction. Am J Cardiol 2014;113:1211–6.

64. Upadhya B, Haykowsky MJ, Eggebeen J, et al. Sarcopenicobesity and the pathogenesis of exercise intolerance in heart failure with preserved ejection fraction. CurrHeart Fail Rep 2015;12:205–14.

65. Packer M, Kitzman DW. Obesity-related heart failure with a preserved ejection fraction. JACC Heart Fail 2018;6:633–9.

66. Alvarez GE, Beske SD, Ballard TP, et al. Sympathetic neural activation in visceral obesity. Circulation 2002;106:2533–6.

67. Lim K, Burke SL, Head GA. Obesity-related hypertension and the role of insulin and leptin in high-fat-fed rabbits. Hypertension 2013;61:628–34.

68. Machleidt F, Simon P, Krapalis AF, et al. Experimental hyperleptinemia acutely increases vasoconstrictory sympathetic nerve activity in healthy humans. J ClinEndocrinolMetab 2013;98:491–6.

69. Sweeney G. Cardiovascular effects of leptin. Nat Rev Cardiol 2010;7:22–9.

70. Rajapurohitam V, Javadov S, Purdham DM, et al. An autocrine role for leptin in mediating the cardiomyocyte hypertrophic effects of angiotensin II and endothelin-1. JMolCellCardiol 2006;41:265–74.

71. Faxén UL, Hage C, Andreasson A, et al. HFpEF and HFrEF exhibit different phenotypes as assessed by leptin and adiponectin. Int J Cardiol 2017;228:709–16.

72. Solomon SD, Zile M, Pieske B, et al. The angiotensin receptor neprilysin inhibitor LCZ696 in heart failure with preserved ejection fraction: a phase 2 double-blind randomised controlled trial. Lancet 2012;380:1387–95.

73. Solomon SD, McMurray JJV, Anand IS, et al. Angiotensin–neprilysin inhibition in heart failure with preserved ejection fraction. N Engl J Med 2019;381(17):1609–20.

74. Obokata M, Kane GC, Reddy YNV, et al. Role of diastolic stress testing in the evaluation for heart

failure with preserved ejection fraction: a simultaneous invasive-echocardiographic study. Circulation 2017;135:825–38.

75. Rider OJ, Ntusi N, Bull SC, et al. Improvements in ECG accuracy for diagnosis of left ventricular hypertrophy in obesity. Heart 2016;102:1566–72.

76. Al-Murshedi S, Hogg P, England A. Relationship between body habitus and image quality and radiation dose in chest X-ray examinations: a phantom study. Phys Med 2019;57:65–71.

77. Sin DD, Jones RL, Paul Man SF. Obesity is a risk factor for dyspnea but not for airflow obstruction. Arch Intern Med 2002;162:1477–81.

78. Larsson SC, Burgess S, Ba M, et al. Body mass index and body composition in relation to 14 CV conditions in UK Biobank. EurHeart J 2020;41:221–6.

79. Ponikowski P, Voors AA, Anker SD, et al. 2016 ESC Guidelines for the diagnosis and treatment of acute and chronic heart failure. EurHeart J 2016;37: 2129–200.

80. Zaphiriou A, Robb S, Murray-Thomas T, et al. The diagnostic accuracy of plasma BNP and NTproBNP in patients referred from primary care with suspected heart failure: Results of the UK natriuretic peptide study. Eur J Heart Fail 2005;7: 537–41.

81. Fuat A, Murphy JJ, Hungin APS, et al. The diagnostic accuracy and utility of a B-type natriuretic peptide test in a community population of patients with suspected heart failure. Br J Gen Pract 2006; 56:327–33.

82. Yamamoto K, Burnett JC, Bermudez EA, et al. Clinical criteria and biochemical markers for the detection of systolic dysfunction. J Card Fail 2000;6: 194–200.

83. Mehra MR, Uber PA, Park MH, et al. Obesity and suppressed B-type natriuretic peptide levels in heart failure. J Am CollCardiol 2004;43:1590–5.

84. McCord J, Mundy BJ, Hudson MP, et al. Relationship between obesity and B-type natriuretic peptide levels. Arch Intern Med 2004;164:2247–52.

85. Wang TJ, Larson MG, Levy D, et al. Impact of obesity on plasma natriuretic peptide levels. Circulation 2004;109:594–600.

86. Chang AY, Abdullah SM, Jain T, et al. Associations among androgens, estrogens, and natriuretic peptides in young women. observations from the dallas heart study. J Am CollCardiol 2007;49:109–16.

87. Khan AM, Cheng S, Magnusson M, et al. Cardiac natriuretic peptides, obesity, and insulin resistance: Evidence from two community-based studies. J ClinEndocrinolMetab 2011;96:3242–9.

88. Mueller C, McDonald K, de Boer RA, et al. Heart Failure Association of the European Society of Cardiology practical guidance on the use of natriuretic peptide concentrations. Eur J Heart Fail 2019;21: 715–31.

89. Myhre PL, Vaduganathan M, Claggett BL, et al. Association of natriuretic peptides with cardiovascular prognosis in heart failure with preserved ejection fraction: secondary analysis of the TOPCAT randomized clinical trial. JAMACardiol 2018; 02115:1–6.

90. Maisel A, Mueller C, Nowak R, et al. Mid-region pro-hormone markers for diagnosis and prognosis in acute dyspnea. results from the bach (biomarkers in acute heart failure) trial. J Am CollCardiol 2010;55:2062–76.

91. Shah RV, Truong QA, Gaggin HK, et al. Mid-regional pro-atrial natriuretic peptide and pro-adrenomedullin testing for the diagnostic and prognostic evaluation of patients with acute dyspnoea. EurHeart J 2012;33:2197–205.

92. Baessler A, Strack C, Rousseva E, et al. Growth-differentiation factor-15 improves reclassification for the diagnosis of heart failure with normal ejection fraction in morbid obesity. Eur J Heart Fail 2012;14:1240–8.

93. Nagueh SF, Smiseth OA, Appleton CP, et al. Recommendations for the evaluation of left ventricular diastolic function by echocardiography: an update from the American Society of Echocardiography and the European Association of Cardiovascular Imaging. J Am SocEchocardiogr 2016;29:277–314.

94. Lancellotti P, Galderisi M, Edvardsen T, et al. Echo-Doppler estimation of left ventricular filling pressure: results of themulticentre EACVI Euro-Filling study. EurHeart J CardiovascImaging 2017;18:961–8.

95. Balaney B, Medvedofsky D, Mediratta A, et al. Invasive validation of the echocardiographic assessment of left ventricular filling pressures using the 2016 diastolic guidelines: head-to-head comparison with the 2009 guidelines. J Am SocEchocardiogr 2018;31:79–88.

96. Sato K, Grant ADM, Negishi K, et al. Reliability of updated left ventricular diastolic function recommendations in predicting elevated left ventricular filling pressure and prognosis. Am Heart J 2017; 189:28–39.

97. De Simone G, Devereux RB, Roman MJ, et al. Relation of obesity and gender to left ventricular hypertrophy in normotensive and hypertensive adults. Hypertension 1994;23:600–6.

98. Picano E, Scali MC, Ciampi Q, et al. Lung ultrasound for the cardiologist. JACCCardiovascImaging 2018;11:1692–705.

99. Martindale JL, Wakai A, Collins SP, et al. Diagnosing acute heart failure in the emergency department: a systematic review and meta-analysis. AcadEmerg Med 2016;23:223–42.

100. Platz E, Merz A, Silverman M, et al. Association between lung ultrasound findings and invasive exercise haemodynamics in patients with undifferentiated dyspnoea. ESC Heart Fail 2019;6(1):202–7.

101. Reddy YNV, Obokata M, Wiley B, et al. The haemo-dynamic basis of lung congestion during exercise in heart failure with preserved ejection fraction. EurHeart J 2019;40(45):3721–30.

102. Palazzuoli A, Ruocco G, Beltrami M, et al. Combined use of lung ultrasound, B-type natriuretic peptide, and echocardiography for outcome prediction in patients with acute HFrEF and HFpEF. Clin Res Cardiol 2018;107:586–96.

103. Mikhalkova D, Holman SR, Jiang H, et al. Bariatric surgery–induced cardiac and lipidomic changes in obesity-related heart failure with preserved ejection fraction. Obesity (Silver Spring) 2018;26:284–90.

104. Adamson PB, Abraham WT, Bourge RC, et al. Wireless pulmonary artery pressure monitoring guides management to reduce decompensation in heart failure with preserved ejection fraction. Circ Heart Fail 2014;7:935–44.

105. McMurray JJV, Solomon SD, Inzucchi SE, et al. Dapagliflozin patients with heart failure and reduced ejection fraction. N Engl J Med 2019;381(21):1995–2008.

106. Inzucchi SE, Zinman B, Wanner C, et al. SGLT-2 inhibitors and cardiovascular risk: Proposed pathways and review of ongoing outcome trials. DiabVasc Dis Res 2015;12:90–100.

107. Gustafsson F, Kragelund CB, Torp-Pedersen C, et al. Effect of obesity and being overweight on long-term mortality in congestive heart failure: Influence of left ventricular systolic function. EurHeart J 2005;26:58–64.

108. Lavie CJ, Alpert MA, Arena R, et al. Impact of obesity and the obesity paradox on prevalence and prognosis in heart failure. JACC Heart Fail 2013;1:93–102.

109. Padwal R, Mcalister FA, Mcmurray JJV, et al. The obesity paradox in heart failure patients with preserved versus reduced ejection fraction: A meta-analysis of individual patient data. Int J Obes 2014;38:1110–4.

Moving?

Make sure your subscription moves with you!

To notify us of your new address, find your **Clinics Account Number** (located on your mailing label above your name), and contact customer service at:

Email: journalscustomerservice-usa@elsevier.com

800-654-2452 (subscribers in the U.S. & Canada)
314-447-8871 (subscribers outside of the U.S. & Canada)

Fax number: 314-447-8029

Elsevier Health Sciences Division
Subscription Customer Service
3251 Riverport Lane
Maryland Heights, MO 63043

*To ensure uninterrupted delivery of your subscription,
please notify us at least 4 weeks in advance of move.

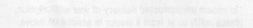

Printed and bound by CPI Group (UK) Ltd, Croydon, CR0 4YY

03/10/2024

01040307-0010